The No-hassle Protein Diet
The Unbalanced Diet Approach
to a Slimmer You

Tran Tien Chanh MD PhD
in collaboration with Béatrice Bottet

The No-hassle Protein Diet
The Unbalanced Diet Approach to a Slimmer You

Translated from the French by Anke Guérin
www.eurotranslationusa.com

Published by
Ideal Protein

ISBN: 2-912160-17-0
© Éditions Ideal Protein
178 Jean-Proulx, Suite 202
Tel.: 1.866.314.4447
Graphic Design: Orage Communication
Printed by DMI – Documents Majemta Inc.

To the mother of my children

CONTENTS

Introduction 13

Chapter 1
Figure, Weight, Where's the Standard?....................15

Chapter 2
How the Method Came About.................................23

Chapter 3
Getting it Right...29

Chapter 4
Eating Better ≠ Weight Loss..................................33

Chapter 5
Weight Loss is Not a Natural Process.....................37

Chapter 6
Ditch Those Ineffective Diets.................................43

Chapter 7
Ketosis: The Why and How of Weight Loss............51

Chapter 8
The Protein Diet, Tried and True............................57

Chapter 9
The Protein Diet Phases...63

Chapter 10
Stabilization..73

Chapter 11
An Easy Maintenance Diet.....................................81

Chapter 12
Why Complex Carbohydrates in the Evening?......................87

Chapter 13
Getting Back on Track 93

Chapter 14
They're All Against You...99

Chapter 15
Exercise, the Finishing Touch................................107

Chapter 16
Recap...115

Chapter 17
Frequently Asked Questions...................................119

Conclusion...129

APPENDICES

Appendix 1:
The Big Three: Proteins, Carbohydrates and Fats 133

Appendix 2:
Understanding the Glycemic Index 145

Appendix 3:
GI: Your Last Diet! 149

Bibliography..153

INTRODUCTION

Well, well, if it isn't another weight-loss book. Hasn't the subject been beaten to death already? Going by the print media, among other indicators, the opposite seems to be true. Slimming down is a matter of health and, in the minds of most women, it's also a matter of beauty. And when it comes to beauty, women's opinions are often shaped by a multitude of factors, such as the shifting vision of beauty over the centuries and women's desire to attain an ideal that is not always of their choosing.

Whatever the case, excess weight is definitely a handicap. Overweight individuals understandably feel bad. Losing weight is not all that difficult, but keeping it off – especially in the long term – is.

That's where the hugely popular protein diet excels. Is it just another fad or a real solution to weight problems?

At a time when everyone is taking credit for this or that protocol, it's worth mentioning that the protein diet – whose idea was developed by Blackburn in the United States in the mid-1970s – was launched in France in the early 1980s and has helped put that country at the forefront of weight loss.

The protein diet has been around for some thirty years and was initially offered to select individuals. We will attempt to demonstrate in this book that nature has made the protein diet THE true weight-loss solution.

Not a single incident has been ascribed to the protein diet since it has been used in Europe by well-informed physicians. Countless practitioners have their patients follow the protein diet successfully. It's a medical method.

Critics who were unfamiliar with the diet's features had a field day. After all, talk about dietetics has focused on a single consensus for decades. Is the consensus any different at the dawn of the third millennium than it was in the 1950s? Hasn't it become a tad old-fashioned and doesn't it need a good updating?

Protein is not an end in itself, but a means or a tool. And like any tool, you must know how to use it.

If you were handed a Stradivarius, but didn't know how to play it, would you say: "The violin? Oh no, I'm against it…"? Would you say that music is stupid? No. You'd learn how to play the violin, see what happens when you know how to play it and then, and only then, would you pass judgement on music, violins in general and the Stradivarius in particular.

The protein diet is an ideal weight-loss instrument, provided you know how to use it.

What's the ideal way to lose weight? Eating better, or more nutritionally, is a good way to maintain a healthy weight, but it won't result in weight loss. You could eat less. Eating less is definitely necessary, but it's not sufficient.

When you lose weight, you lose fat. And when you lose fat, you unfortunately also lose protein mass or muscles (protein mass also includes the internal organs: the heart, liver, kidneys, etc.). Weight loss while retaining muscle mass implies that lost protein must be compensated for by a calculated protein intake as part of a low-calorie, time-limited diet.

Ideally, dieters lose fat without losing any muscle and maintain their new weight by eating a nutritional diet.

Those same dieters will lose weight more quickly and keep the pounds off longer, because after reading this book they'll understand why they accumulated fat and learn how to lose it. That should keep them from backsliding, help them stay on track and make them more aware of changes.

You find those extra pounds annoying and would love to have a perfect figure, but you hesitate because of the perceived difficulty of losing weight. All you need is willpower. Your efforts will yield results, with no risk of "yo-yoing".

1 Figure, Weight, Where's the Standard?

The beauty of the human body, especially the female body, has always been shaped by opinions that are often contradictory. A woman must be able to procreate, meet expectations (morals, customs, virtues, good manners, modesty) and be pretty in her eyes and in those of the future father of her children. That's quite a conformity-oriented order to fill!

Beauty or Conformity?

Has a woman's body changed significantly over the centuries? Its height certainly has, as each passing century has seen women's height increase by an inch or so. However, the answer to the above question is not as clear when it comes to the distribution of fat and diverse morphologies. Uniformity, or even conformity, is an illusion that continues to boost the sales of companies specializing in external beauty (fashion, cosmetics) and internal beauty (diets, body sculpting). There have always been lanky and short women, thin and voluptuous women, curvaceous and lean women, soft and muscular women.

When the idealized image of a woman's body is evoked, there is no doubt. Whether that image is held by men or women, the female body has undergone random and absurd changes and modifications.

If a woman's body does not spontaneously conform to what is deemed gorgeous at the time, we'll help it conform with all kinds of coercion ranging from support garments to social pressure. In most cases, fashion – the fantastical and idealized representation of the female body – has endeavoured to highlight the reproductive functions, like the nourishing breasts and voluptuous hips associated with the full-term pregnancies of prehistoric Venuses. The West has been providing an acceptable representation of this for a thousand years.

Fashion, the Standardizer of the Female Figure

In the Middle Ages, the female figure had to be tall and curved. The ideal female figure featured small, firm, white breasts, tilted hips and a rounded stomach. Even young girls strived to look pregnant. An attractive woman was one that evoked a maternal image. Women in the Middle Ages were not encumbered with tight, uncomfortable clothing and had a flexible, relaxed posture – even slouched compared to what would come in future centuries.

That would soon all change.

The Renaissance was not a time of progress for women. Clothing restricted their movements and showed them off. Freedom and ease of movement had gone out the window. Women had to submit. To be pretty, attractive and meet expectations (from attire to modesty), they more or less wore a straitjacket: a cone-shaped, hard and stiff corset – the precursor of the corset as we think of it – which constricted the waist, flattened the chest, chaffed skin, made breathing difficult and diminished appetite.

The Renaissance marked the beginning of standardized figures, without giving a single thought to diversity and the very nature of the female body and to the detriment of free movement. The corset would be around for centuries.

At the time of Henry VI, however, being overweight was in style, and newspapers of the time were filled with tips on how to gain weight because "being skinny is hideous". How times changed.

Corsets were in style for five centuries. It wasn't until World War I that women finally freed themselves from tight-fitting, unnatural attire.

Social Pressure, Another Form of Coercion

Nowadays, women want to be free. Free to dress as they see fit, free to walk in long strides, free to take part in sports, free to be accountable to no one. They own their body, demand that it be theirs and are proud of it. But are they free of the requirements of public opinion that incessantly dictates everything to which they must conform and the image they must convey?

The answer is, obviously, no. Modern women are as submitted to conventions, conformisms and coercion as were their grandmothers, great-grandmothers and ancestors. The difference is that most restrictions are no longer visible. The corset may be gone, but women must be at a specific weight for their height and shed a few more pounds because they don't want to look ridiculous at the beach. They must have shapely buttocks and a flat stomach, be slender, and have perky breasts that are neither too big nor too small. Women must fit into a mold again.

Men, too, have an ideal image to live up to, which makes them ever more conscious of their figure, but they face less demanding social and esthetic pressures.

Would You Gain Ten Pounds to Fit a Standard?

Beauty criteria have resulted in implicit laws that are far more stringent than any legislation. You must, you must not, you have to… Standardization is a heavy burden and those who follow it to the letter lack perspective, critical sense and even common sense. Let me give you an example.

A patient made an appointment with me. She weighs about 80 kilograms (180 pounds). She came along with a friend and asked if her friend could sit in on the consultation, which I gladly agreed to.

I asked the patient: "How much would you like to weigh?"

Before she could answer my question, her friend intervened.

"You should weigh 56 kilograms (123 pounds)."

I turned to the friend and said: "Is that so? Why do you say that?"

"Well", the friend replied, "she's 1.66 metres tall. You take the number of centimetres in excess of one metre, subtract ten and obtain your ideal weight: 66 minus 10 equals 56 kilograms."

The friend had an outdated method of calculating ideal weight, but that is neither here nor there… This incredible theoretician was also a model. I asked her a few questions.

"So, how much do you weigh?"

"I weigh 56 kilograms," she replied proudly.

"And how tall are you?"

"1.76 metres."

"So, if I go by your reasoning, you should weigh 66

kilograms."

"What!" she exclaimed.

"Sure, if you subtract ten from the number of centimetres in excess of one metre, you get 66. Would you be willing to gain ten kilograms to meet your standard?"

"Absolutely not," she said, "especially since I feel so good at my current weight."

She was probably referring to the Duchess of Windsor who proclaimed, "You can never be too rich or too thin".

"If you don't want to adhere to the standard, why impose it on your friend?" I asked.

That's the whole issue. Although such criteria give a rough idea of how much you should weigh, they must be handled with extreme caution in order to avoid aberrant situations that may lead to medical conditions or psychological disorders.

What is Normality Exactly?

All dieters must think there are inequalities, genetic injustices and different tastes, but they must never forget that there is no one standard for beauty, weight or a figure, but rather different normalities.

Is it more normal to have straight or curly hair? Is it more normal to have blue or brown eyes? Must a man be between 5'9" and 6'1" tall in order to be "handsome"? Must a woman's bra size be at least a pretty 34C? Normality sometimes deviates significantly from the criteria and rules by which everyone should abide.

Nutritionists have no absolute standard for normality. Normality is feeling good and being in good health, which is not bad at all. It's not a series of abstract numbers or absurd dictates. Fashion can be terrifying at times and is often created by designers who take into account the type of figure they find alluring – androgynous or, to be very specific, even android as opposed to gynoid (more on that later). Such fashion, which is suitable only for a small percentage of women and far removed from female body shapes, is much more dictatorial than health imperatives.

In Search of the Perfect Figure

As a physician, I refuse to trap my patients in such a system of rules, criteria, obligations and dietary restrictions. Besides, more often than not, those who come to see me about their weight problems are perfectly clear-headed.

When I ask them: "What do you think is your ideal weight?" most give me a very reasonable answer based on their height, lifestyle, and life history (age, pregnancies...). Very rarely do they have exaggerated weight-loss expectations.

That is not the case with gynoid women, who have small breasts and a large lower body characterized by wide, curvaceous hips, visible saddlebags and a prominent stomach. Since they are naturally heavy on the bottom and put on weight below the waistline, they are overweight (sometimes just a little) and take it badly. They have a double body image: normal for the upper body and dysmorphic for the lower body, as if it were someone else's.

They consider themselves victims of an injustice. So much so that they have difficulty rationally explaining how much weight they should lose and always overestimate by how much they are overweight. For example, they'll say that they are 20 pounds overweight when they need to lose only eight pounds. They think that if they lose more weight, their lower body will be thinner.

Any weight problem must be put into perspective. When a gynoid woman is at a normal weight or needs to shed only a few pounds, a diet will not eliminate the inequality between the upper and lower body. It will improve her figure, but it won't transform it, leaving her hungry for perfection.

People with a gynoid body might be eternally unsatisfied and end up on a permanent diet.

So, the work to be done has nothing to do with a diet and everything to do with accepting the weight problem or putting it into perspective. Any diet can result in weight loss, but no diet can tackle the entirely different problem that is body dysmorphic disorder, or an obsession with one's own appearance and never being satisfied with it despite one's best efforts.

Nowadays, everyone knows that you follow a diet for health reasons.

Food has become much fatter and sweeter over the last century and even more so in the past fifty years. All that fat and sugar is harmful to health.

Obesity is unattractive and tires the heart. Excess sugar and fat leads to diabetes. Therefore, shedding those extra pounds is more a matter of health than fashion. Let's be more sensible than our predecessors by ridding our bodies of excess weight and not dreaming of having the atypical figure of a model.

2 How the Method Came About

An idea or a method is often borne of an observation, sometimes unexpected, that corroborates theories or research. The idea of putting overweight patients on the protein diet – a known, but somewhat abandoned procedure – came to me from sports.

Behind the Sports Scene

After being a high-level athlete (a former champion university boxer) and Thai boxing instructor, I embarked on a career as a sports physician. I worked with boxers, champion triathletes, dancers, marathon runners…

Why would athletes need to lose weight? Most are not fat because of their training and carefully calibrated diet. However, their weight can fluctuate and athletes who want to remain in their category must keep a close eye on their weight.

Athletes do not take care of themselves any which way, and they don't lose weight any which way either. Firstly, they cannot be given amphetamines, which are appetite suppressants and stimulants, eliminate fatigue and… produce positive anti-doping tests. Secondly, athletes may need to lose weight, but they definitely want to retain their muscle mass. Obviously, a diet must not result in both fat and muscle loss.

For example, a boxer slated for a major fight in two or three months must prepare by training now. What does he do to control his weight, or rather what did he do up until a few years ago to reach the right weight for his category? During the days leading up to the fight, he worked on dehydration: sauna, Turkish baths, wearing a raincoat while training or even turning up his car's heater to maximum. The more affluent boxers took a more serious, medically supervised approach, but the principle remained dehydration. As a result, on the day of the fight, they all had deficiencies in trace elements and mineral salts, particularly potassium. Potassium is involved in muscle contraction (a potassium deficiency causes muscle cramps). Since they had lost water and mineral salts, they entered the fighting ring lighter, but weakened to the point that their two months of preparation had been wiped out.

It turned out that it was far more effective to put boxers who needed to lose five to ten pounds on a protein diet. After they lost the fat but no muscle mass, they were told to eat slow sugars to ensure they would be in optimal shape on the day of the fight and have all the energy they needed.

The protein diet, once reserved for extremely obese hospitalized individuals under close medical supervision, was extended to athletes and recommended more to men than to women. Today the opposite is true: more overweight women than men follow the protein diet in order to lose excess weight.

Can Everyone Benefit from the Protein Diet?

At the time, I had two types of patients to whom I applied different protocols: an athletic clientele that went on the protein diet and an office clientele for whom I prescribed a typical, supposedly balanced, low-calorie diet.

After some time, I realized that the first group of patients obtained the expected results almost consistently, without being fatigued and while staying in excellent shape. The second group of "ordinary" patients was hungry, gave up, gained back the weight – yo-yoing – was tired and showed all the signs of diminished energy levels.

So I started to use the athlete protocol for patients who, I thought, would benefit from it. The results were so interesting that they raised the following question: couldn't the method be used for all overweight individuals (except where absolutely contraindicated)?

Among the criticisms levelled against the protein diet, the following is the most frequent: Isn't it like using a sledgehammer to kill a mosquito?

Why use longer, more tiresome methods that yield poor results when there's a method that consistently works and never leads to any medical conditions? He who has more can do less. If seriously obese individuals and athletes can benefit from the protein diet, why can't people with just a few pounds to lose also benefit from it, especially since it is safe and fits well with family and professional responsibilities?

Anyone who is overweight suffers, and the suffering is not necessarily proportional to the number of pounds to be lost. You do not suffer less because you have fewer pounds to lose.

You feel down and are unhappy with your physique, and that suffering can easily be relieved. Could you bear to be told: "You only have a few pounds to lose, so there's no point in using the best weight-loss method"? That's ridiculous.

Do not Systemize

I now use the protein diet method for most patients who consult me about weight loss. It's a relatively short-term diet that must be coupled with a stabilization phase; however, the protein diet is not always the starting point.

In fact, some people are overweight because they eat to excess and must first be encouraged to eat less.

Most people do not overeat. Many of my patients eat poorly, but not necessarily too much. They think they have tried everything; they've tried out various diets and systems, and they just can't shed those extra pounds. Since these people need more than a balanced diet, I attack the problem head on with the protein diet, because not only does it promote weight loss, but it also helps to improve the health of the pancreas.

Ketosis (more on this term later) induced by the protein diet corrects the pancreas' metabolism. When the pancreas is not functioning properly, it causes too much sugar to be absorbed and fat to be stored. Once the way the pancreas responds to food has been corrected, it functions so well that cravings for sweets disappear and the body functions as it should have all along.

The protein diet method has other advantages: it does not tire the body, it does not melt away muscle mass, it is used over the short term so that it's easier to respect restrictions and it does not result in the rebound effect or yo-yoing (as long as you change any bad food habits you may have). Nor does it cause depression. On the contrary, patients feel good, energetic and even blissful. All of this is achieved without the use of any medication whatsoever. Moreover, the protein diet is entirely physiological or natural and contains no chemical compounds.

The method's very principle has benefits for everyone. Patients who have lost excess weight by following the protein diet only have good things to say about it. Once you understand the protein diet's principles, you'll see how simple and effective it is.

3 Getting it Right

What criteria are used to evaluate weight? Obviously, you can't go by the advice and pictures in magazines and even less by the images of bombshells served up by the fashion industry that would have us believe that models and top models are the epitome of beauty and the perfect objects of desire.

Top Models are a Bad Example

Young models, whose measurements are common knowledge, do not represent normal women. In fact, their measurements are very different from those of the standard population and their BMI (see below) is significantly lower.

Clothes look better on tall and slender figures. And let's not forget that many magazine photos are touched up in order to modify proportions or shading. So stop basing yourself on the measurements of these models in order to determine your desired or right weight.

Body Mass Index (BMI)

You may already be familiar with the term Body Mass Index (BMI), a calculation that evaluates your height-to-weight ratio to determine if you are at a healthy body weight. It has a rather wide range.

BMI, also known as the Quetelet Index, has replaced other evaluations and formulae. It is now considered entirely reliable and is used by all nutritionists, dieticians and other health care specialists.

Here's how to calculate your BMI:

Divide your weight (in pounds) by your height (in inches) squared and multiply the quotient (result) by 703. If your BMI is between 20 and 25, your weight-to-height ratio is normal and you have no excess weight that poses a health risk.

Example: You are 5'3" (63 inches) tall and weigh 126 pounds.

$$\text{Your BMI is:} \quad \frac{126}{63 \times 63} \quad \times\ 703 \quad = 22.3$$

With a BMI of 22.3, your weight is ideal.

If you were taller and weighed less, your BMI would be between 18.5 and 20, which is a little low (you are too thin), but there would be no health risks. However, if your BMI was less than 18.5, you'd have to gain a few pounds. (Most models have a BMI of 16 to 18...)

If your BMI was between 25 and 30, you'd have reason to be alarmed, because you'd be overweight and your health would be at risk. Obviously, the higher your BMI, the more obese you are and the more your health is at risk. If your BMI was over 30, you'd be dangerously obese and have to go on a diet under the guidance of a nutritionist. Some people have a BMI greater than 40. They are pathologically obese, have numerous health problems and must obviously lose weight and be closely monitored.

4 Eating Better ≠ Weight Loss

A question must be properly formulated before it can be answered. Nutritionally speaking, have we always been asking the right question? What exactly is a diet? Must you eat better? Must you eat less?

Up until now, all methods that restricted caloric intake and that were supplemented by medication (diuretics, amphetamines or thyroid extracts) have always proven dangerous without exception. The only totally safe method is one that has no active ingredients and that relies solely on the body's physiological principles. That describes the protein diet.

It should be stated from the outset that protein is not an active ingredient that promotes weight loss, and that supplemental proteins are used to protect muscles and the body's protein mass.

Eating Poorly = Weight Gain

Eating poorly leads to weight gain. It's a no-brainer. We all know what eating poorly is: too many sweets and fats; gourmandizing; chocolate and candies to ward off stress; ready-made meals and take-home salads drowning in mayonnaise because you didn't have time to cook or do the groceries; an aperitif and peanuts; munching while watching TV; stopping at a bakery to pick up a chocolate doughnut because you're feeling a little hungry.

Advertising, especially television advertising, encourages us to eat an incredible range of carbohydrate-containing products: milk desserts, cakes, sodas, fruit juices… These incessant inducements or temptations discourage those who want to lose weight. They also create a sort of perpetual conflict: I must not eat it, but I sure do feel like it. All that tension caused by pleasure versus duty (a duty to diet in this case) only adds to our stressed-out lives.

Eating poorly causes weight gain, and unfortunately the opposite is not always true: eating well does not necessarily make you lose weight. What a shame!

You want to lose weight because you overate or because of your irregular metabolism. You naturally think that you'll have to eat better and less to lose those pounds you packed on.

Eating less is a necessary but insufficient condition. Some people drop down to their right weight as soon as they eat less, like a delighted young woman who explains to her friends that she just lost 15 pounds: "And it wasn't even hard. All I did was cut out the sodas and fries for two weeks."

If you haven't had any coke or fries for a long time and if you already eat wisely, you have every reason to be jealous. Some people can eat what they want and even more and stay as thin as a toothpick.

A young man who was thin as a rail, asked me: "Why shouldn't I put butter and chocolate spread on my chocolate croissant?" Genetics can be so unfair…

Everyone who wants you to slim down will tell you that the alternative is to eat better. It's a defendable theory.

Eating Well ≠ Weight Loss

Everyone thinks that eating well means eating a more balanced diet. A balanced diet is synonymous with no change, a state of equilibrium. Where there is balance, there is no change. That's exactly what you don't want if you want to lose weight!

If I put a patient on a balanced diet, she won't gain weight, but she won't lose any either: her weight is stable.

Now here's a surprising principle to keep in mind if you want to lose weight:

> • **If you want to lose weight, you must take the unbalanced diet approach.**

If you want to lose weight and fat, you'll have to eliminate something. And when you eliminate something from your diet, it's deficient. Obviously, if your diet is deficient you're not eating better. You're eating differently.

Nutritional deficiency! A diet that intentionally lacks something! You shudder at the idea!

A deficient diet is quite acceptable under the following conditions:

- the unbalanced diet must not be dangerous;
- the deficiency must be of limited duration and have a beginning and an end;
- the deficiency must be useful and effective.

That's why an intentionally unbalanced, deficient diet must absolutely be recommended and monitored by a nutritionist, because you don't want to lose weight and cause a medical condition and a vitamin and mineral salt deficiency.

Furthermore, this treatment imposes sacrifices, because you'll have to say good-bye to dinners with friends, gourmandizing and tasty treats. In addition to making you lose weight, this treatment, like any other treatment, has benefits that will be examined later, as well as some drawbacks.

Keeping it Straight

By now you've come across quite a few terms: lose weight, shed pounds, balanced, unbalanced, dietetics, eat better, eat less.

If you want to understand the process thoroughly and consequently lose weight better, remember this:

- **Weight loss conflicts with the concept of eating better.**

In summary, dieters have two opposite approaches or contracts:

- an approach that introduces an imbalance for a limited period of time in order to bring about **weight loss** safely;

- a dietetic approach based on eating better that aims to **maintain an ideal weight** and that may (and should) have no time limit.

Remember this fundamental concept. Once you have made the distinction between the two approaches, you'll be able to follow the treatment happily and enthusiastically.

- **Never confuse the concept of weight loss with the concept of dietetics.**

5 Weight Loss is Not a Natural Process

Weight loss is not a natural process for humans (or animals for that matter), hence the need to introduce the concept of imbalance which goes against our healthy concepts of food.

From the time of the first hominids up until the *Homo sapiens sapiens* that we have become, we have never been programmed to lose weight. Nothing in our physiology, apart from *ketosis*, is designed for weight loss.

The Human Body is not Designed to Lose Fat

We eat to store energy and build up energy reserves and not to decrease them. Humans are the only animals that eat for pleasure. Adipocytes, fat cells distributed throughout the body based on gender, store fat as a survival strategy to see us through times of famine.

There are two types of fat distribution in women: android (apple-shaped body; upper body fat) and gynoid (pear-shaped body; lower body fat).

Gynoid women tend to put on weight around the hips, thighs, and lower abdomen, which helps them reach full-term pregnancies safely and breast feed. In gynoid women, fat is released slowly: the survival of the human race depends on it. Women must have fat reserves that can be used over the very long term and released very slowly.

In men, fat cells are concentrated in the shoulders, chest and upper body. This fat can be used rapidly during a brief, one-time, physically demanding event, like hunting a mammoth.

Anyone who was able to store fat proved they were doing well. Should they have been unable to do so, the situation would have been dire indeed.

These predispositions, which go back to time immemorial, are now much more of a hindrance for weight-conscious women than men. While men are able to lose weight fairly easily, a woman's body is reluctant to empty its fat reserves. In fact, it only empties those reserves when it has no choice and is reminded of the ancient reasons why fat is stored in saddlebags: severe famines and interminable food shortages.

Consequently, the body must be tricked into thinking there is a famine. That's why an imbalance or a deficiency must be introduced. Once ample food is again available, the body will have to be taught not to store fat and that's the hardest part.

Nature never planned that man would have to eat and lose weight at the same time. Weight loss is unnatural.

Weight gain is influenced by hormones. We gain weight in the fall in preparation for the winter; we gain weight when we are under stress... Our body has a deeply rooted seasonal physiology of which we are totally unaware, but that watches over us on the off chance... So, it's a good idea to shed those excess pounds after the winter.

An upset patient said to me: "It's horrible, doctor, I've gained 65 pounds in thirty years. When I was young, I weighed 120 pounds and now I weigh 185!"

It's not extremely unusual for an individual to gain 65 pounds between the age of 20 and menopause. In fact, it's quite common. This particular patient may be upset about her weight gain, but it's not necessarily pathological. She has no medical condition or illness and her tests are normal. Could you imagine the opposite: a 120-pound patient who lost 65 pounds in thirty years and who now weighs a mere 55 pounds? That's just unthinkable. Nature planned for weight gain; spontaneous weight loss is unnatural.

How the Body Stores Fat

The pancreas is the main organ responsible for converting sugars into fat and storing fat in the body (fats and sugars converted into fat).

The pancreas, an endocrine gland, produces the hormone insulin when stimulated by simple or complex carbohydrates. So, you must eat carbohydrates in order to produce insulin.

Insulin has two roles:

- lower blood sugar (a regulatory role); and

- store fat in the body (insulin is the hormone that stimulates lipogenesis, i.e. the production of fat).

When you eat sugar, the pancreas produces insulin in order to lower your blood sugar.

Unfortunately, your pancreas can go into overdrive, producing too much insulin for the amount of sugar consumed. The excess insulin causes your blood sugar to plunge rapidly. As a result, your body experiences a carbohydrate deficiency as it were and demands more sugar. This is called a hypoglycemic episode. Your craving for something sweet is so strong that you almost feel sick. There is also "normal" hypoglycemia: those little hunger pangs you feel at 11 a.m. or towards the end of the afternoon.

And so begins a vicious circle: excess sugar causes excess insulin production, which causes excessive sugar consumption and so on. Insulin betrays you, rapidly converting sugar into fat and storing it, because excess insulin naturally promotes fat storage. It's truly a vicious circle.

The pancreas is like a furnace that's out of control. And when your pancreas is out of control, you tire more quickly. Hypoglycemics tire quickly through no fault of their own and are also more predisposed to prediabetes and diabetes.

The Pancreas is the Culprit

The pancreas is the culprit of fat storage. Simple and complex carbohydrates, which do not have pernicious health effects in and of themselves, cause fat to accumulate in the body if the pancreas is in a hyperinsulinemic state.

Of the endocrine glands (like the thyroid, reproductive glands, pituitary gland and adrenal glands), the pancreas is probably upset the most easily and also the easiest to reset. All you need to do is give it a break by cutting off its supply of sugar – the furnace's fuel.

The pancreas is essentially regulated by external stimulation – food that is ingested. However, even when retrained or reset, the pancreas may have a natural tendency to produce too much insulin. Is the situation hopeless? Not necessarily, because a retrained pancreas works better than a non-retrained one. We know how to keep it from going out of control.

What is the difference between a person who tends to store fat and another who burns a lot of fat? Well, it's the proportion of carbohydrates in the diet. More on that later.

There has been much talk of late about "metabolic syndrome" (or Syndrome X), which is characterized by weight gain (especially in and around the abdomen), prediabetes, high blood fat (high level of bad cholesterol or triglycerides) and elevated blood pressure. An individual need not exhibit these four symptoms in order to have metabolic syndrome. Thus, obesity combined with hypertension, diabetes or cholesterol may be a sign of metabolic syndrome.

Metabolic syndrome is actually caused by insulin dysfunction, **either insulin resistance or hyperinsulinism**.

Little is known about metabolic syndrome, a very widespread disorder that affects over 60 million Americans. Generally speaking, 25% of the non-diabetic population has insulin dysfunction and 25% will go on to develop type 2 diabetes (non-insulin-dependent diabetes).

Public Enemy Number One of the Third Millennium

Obesity and metabolic syndrome are one of the leading causes of death in industrialized nations, particularly in North America.

Unfortunately, both are on the rise. Given the magnitude of this phenomenon, physicians and epidemiologists no longer hesitate to sound the alarm and speak of a modern epidemic, the scourge of the 21st century, and even public enemy number one.

It is now known that there is a direct link between obesity and type 2 diabetes, and the onset of "societal" degenerative diseases, such as cardiovascular diseases, cancer, inflammatory diseases and neurovegetative disorders.

Factors Responsible for Obesity and Metabolic Syndrome

- Genetic factors.

- Nutritional causes, such as eating too much fast sugar,

41

refined carbohydrates (refined flours, for example) and saturated fats.

- Behavioural factors, such as a lack of exercise.

Although the "scourge of the 21st century" is worrying, the situation is not hopeless because a remedy is usually discovered years or decades after an epidemic has been identified.

There is real hope in the case of metabolic syndrome. Even if obesity and insulin dysfunction have been termed a real epidemic for only two or three years, the remedy has been around for 15 years already.

And that's good news!

"Insulin resistance occurs when normal insulin activity is weakened and cells do not respond to the insulin "signal" sent by the pancreas. The pancreas produces ever more insulin in order to overcome this decreased activity and maintain blood glucose balance."

Dr. Lukaczer, D. Nutritional Support for Insulin Resistance. ANSR, July 1, 2001.

---

6 Ditch Those Ineffective Diets

Losing weight is very difficult. The very nature of human beings who are designed to store rather than to burn fat runs contrary to weight loss, as does an overactive or malfunctioning pancreas or overwhelming sugar cravings. The only solution is to go on a diet and hope that you won't put the pounds back on.

Everyone says that they quickly regain weight after they've gone on a diet. That's because they've decreased their muscle mass. However, if they had lost weight by decreasing their body fat, the situation would be different.

It Takes More Than Energy Balance

There are countless diets and many are based on scientific theories that hold water. All diets result in weight loss, but none will prevent the return of the lost weight.

Up until now, excess weight has essentially been addressed with the concept of energy balance, resting metabolism and energy expenditure. So it's logical that weight management is based solely on reducing calories and increasing physical activity.

This approach is pertinent but insufficient, because it is based on quantity and does not adequately take account of the fact that overall reduced food intake results in fat and muscle loss. The weight issue is attacked from the wrong angle.

This approach does not take into account metabolism and the role of hormones either. It is because of these two factors that some people can eat what they want and not gain an ounce, while others seem to gain weight just by looking at a pastry shop window. It is also because of these two factors that people do not all respond in the same way biologically or physiologically to identical food intakes.

Diets Never Work More Than Once

All diets are low-calorie diets, but frequently recommended typical "low-calorie" diets virtually always lead to weight gain and to devastating and depressing yo-yoing.

Incidentally, the number of calories in these supposedly balanced diets is no "lower" than, or different from, that in other diets. You consume fewer calories because you're eating less.

What is a "balanced weight-loss diet"? Simply put, a balanced weight-loss diet means eating less of everything: less carbohydrates, protein and fat. The overall amount of food is reduced, while the three categories of foods remain balanced. But remember, you need to take an unbalanced diet approach in order to lose weight…

The problem is that when food intake is reduced, so is the amount of useful and less useful foods. An individual who goes on a low-calorie diet might well end up with a protein, mineral salt, vitamin or trace element deficiency.

The good thing about a typical low-calorie diet or a "balanced, low-calorie diet" is that you definitely lose weight. But there's nothing great about that, because all diets result in weight loss. The bad thing is that you don't always lose the pounds where you want.

Low-calorie diets result in fat and muscle loss. If you go off a low-calorie diet, do you think you'll put back on the fat and the muscle in the same way that you lost them? No way. You'll only put back on the fat. Your muscles melted away along with the fat due to a lack of protein. You've lost muscle mass. Muscles are the body's biggest consumer of calories (incidentally, the heart is a muscle) and the engine that "burns" fuel. The more muscle you have, the more calories you'll burn and vice-versa. It follows that if you reduce your muscle mass, you'll also reduce your energy expenditure at rest. Once you begin to eat normally again, you won't have enough muscle to burn the surplus calories, which will then be stored in your fatty tissue. So you put the weight back on. It's a vicious circle.

Things will not improve as time goes by.

Should you follow the advice of some people and eat a balanced diet? If you want… In fact, I'd say you'd be following a nutritionally deficient diet that results not only in weight and fat loss, but also in muscle loss and despair.

A little reminder: muscle mass (or muscles) is part of lean body mass or protein mass, which includes the muscular system and internal organs, which also burn energy and calories.

The Pounds that Keep on Coming Back

You've lost twenty pounds of fat and muscle and you know that once you go back to eating normally, you'll put those twenty pounds back on, mostly in the form of fat. You'll suddenly be tempted to go on another diet, and so on. The more diets you go on, the less weight you'll lose, since your muscles' ability to burn calories will have shrunk because you have less muscle.

Many patients tell me: "Doctor, I went on a low-calorie diet and it worked well the first time, but I never reached the stabilization phase."

Why doesn't a single patient reach the stabilization phase? Because low-calorie diets do not have a stabilization phase.

The human body is excellent at adapting. There's a deficiency? It adapts, it conserves and it conserves some more. It's like money: the less you have, the less you spend and vice versa. Your body does the same thing (I'll get back to that). It adapts when faced with a long-lasting deficiency, by reducing its needs and slowing down its metabolism. As a result, you'll have to eat less and less to continue to lose weight.

That is obviously an unacceptable solution. Who wants to go through life on ever-more restrictive diets?

The Solution: Lose Fat and Keep Muscle

There is another entirely logical solution: long-lasting weight loss can be achieved by losing fat – after all, that has been the goal ever since the beginning – without affecting your muscles and vital organs.

What must you eliminate in order to lose fat? That's a no-brainer: fats and carbohydrates must be cut out. You'll discover later on in this book that there are simple and complex carbohydrates and that both must be eliminated.

> • **To lose weight, you must not only eliminate the foods that make you gain weight, but also those that keep you from losing weight: this is a fundamental concept.**

We all know that fries and cream puffs will make you gain weight. I don't eat foods that make me gain weight, so I don't gain weight. But I'm not losing any either...

An apple is not fattening, you say.

That's true in a normal situation. But if you're on a protein diet, that apple may keep you from losing weight.

A slice of bread won't make you gain weight, but it'll keep you from losing it.

A plate of rice won't make you gain weight, but it'll keep you from losing it.

A glass of wine won't make you gain weight, but it'll keep you from losing it.

A food that is harmless in a normal situation is no longer harmless in a weight-loss situation. It becomes the enemy, a food that keeps you from losing weight.

When you follow the protein diet, you radically change your situation and must follow the diet's instructions to the letter.

Remember, sugars are eliminated until your pancreas has been given a break and the process that forces your body to draw on its reserves has begun.

When you lose weight, you live off your reserves.

The Protein Diet Principle

The protein diet significantly reduces the amount of calories, but it does not follow the same principles as typical, low-calorie, supposedly balanced diets. More importantly, by regulating the pancreas, the protein diet attacks the weight-gain mechanism head on instead of waiting until the damage has been done.

Its aim is to maintain an optimal protein intake without modifying the amount of mineral salts and vitamins in your diet, while significantly reducing carbohydrate and fat intake.

The diet is based on protein meals of which the number is determined by a nutritionist. The meals, sold in packets, are usually mixed with water, sometimes require cooking and resemble traditional prepared foods: soups, omelettes, hot or cold drinks, purees, etc. These food products are developed so as to provide the necessary amount of proteins, with a minimal amount of calories from sugar and fat.

Let's be clear. The packets will usually say "high-protein food". A protein diet is not a high-protein diet in that you don't eat more protein than your body needs.

As you'll see in Appendix 1, your body needs the fuel provided by carbohydrates and fats to function, but proteins are the essential building blocks for most tissue. Your body is primarily composed of protein: muscles, internal organs, the heart, the liver, kidneys, etc. Proteins play a major or significant role in eyes, bones and skin. Hormones and enzymes are also protein structures.

On average, women need 1.2 g of protein per day per kilogram of ideal body weight and men 1.4 g, to keep their body in shape and enable it to perform all of its functions. These figures depend not only on gender, but also on age and life events (pregnancy or breastfeeding, for example). Although these figures are widely accepted, they are probably greater than actual needs.

A woman who weighs 50 kg needs 60 g of protein per day (1.2 x 50 = 60 g).

Where is she going to find that protein? The answer is obvious: in meat, fish, dairy products and eggs.

Half a small steak weighs 60 grams. Your body would have a hard time functioning on so little, because a 60-gram steak does not contain 60 grams of protein. In fact, every 100 grams of steak contains about 20 grams of protein (17 to 13 grams, depending on the meat).

You'd have to eat 300 grams of steak to get 60 grams of protein!

And those 300 grams of meat also contain 240 grams you don't need, including 30 to 60 grams of fat (less for lean cuts). Obviously, this in no way helps you reduce your carbohydrate and fat intake or your caloric intake for that matter.

The one definite benefit of eating meat is that it contains no carbohydrates. Your body will be forced to draw the energy it needs from the fat that has been stored for some time in your fatty tissue, because that is what fat is for.

This physiological process involves converting your body's fat into fuel. *Ketosis* is the process by which your body turns its fat reserves into energy and *gluconeogenesis* is the process by which it converts the amino acids in its muscles into energy.

Let's focus on the principle. By inducing *ketosis*, the protein diet forces your metabolism to convert fat into "fuel" and melt the fat away.

The problem is that you don't want to lose muscle mass in the process.

Three Sources of Energy

The body, like any other machine, needs energy to function. It has three sources of energy or fuel (more on that later):

- carbohydrates (or sugars);
- lipids (or fats);
- proteins.

These three sources of energy are not all used at once in any order; that would be a tremendous waste. Your body sets priorities.

It burns carbohydrates first for its daily energy needs, as carbohydrates are readily available.

It stores lipids and proteins in its energy reserves and does not draw on them as long as it has fuel (carbohydrates) to meet its energy needs. Why dip into your savings account if you have enough money in your current account?

Your body has fat cells – called adipocytes – and protein cells, including muscle cells, but it has no carbohydrate cells. It stores carbohydrates in the form of glycogen in the liver and muscle cells. The next chapter will shed more light on this.

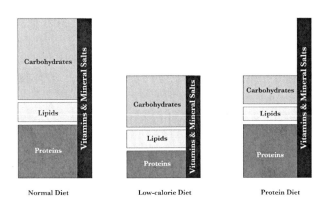

When you're on a balanced, low-calorie diet, you eat a little less of everything, including vitamins, mineral salts, and proteins.

When you follow the protein diet, you cut your carbohydrate and fat intake, while your protein, vitamin and mineral salt intake remains unchanged.

7 Ketosis: The Why and How of Weight Loss

How does the protein diet melt away all the pounds of fat that your body stores by nature? It's not a miracle; it's due to *ketosis*, a word that has come up in earlier chapters.

Fasting Has a Long History

Many cultures advocate some form of fasting or dietary restriction. Their purpose in doing so is not only to inconvenience followers and teach them objectivity, but also to open their minds, as the mystics say, and to distance them from the pleasures of the flesh.

During Advent (the period leading up to Christmas) and Lent (the period leading up to Easter), Christians are to avoid eating animal products and to abstain from overindulgence, although these rules long have been relaxed considerably. Remember? The body gains weight in the fall in preparation for the winter. In the spring, Lent provides an opportunity to eliminate that excess weight.

Ramadan requires Muslims to fast from sunrise to sunset. Since they may break their fast at night, they eat little.

It is said that Buddha spent many years meditating under a banana tree, eating only a grain of rice per day. Many of his followers fast at one time or another. Aren't yogis mainly ascetics?

North American Indians fasted, meditated and took sweat baths individually or collectively prior to an important stage of their life.

Shamans from Siberia to Mexico, *curanderos* (witch doctors-healers) and other medicine men wouldn't even think of going into a trance without fasting, ingesting emetics to induce vomiting and fumigating substances to fully purify themselves.

Gnostics, Cathars and others have all fasted. In Europe, monks, nuns, hermits and cenobites regularly denied themselves much more food than did ordinary believers.

Why Deny Yourself Food Voluntarily?

Why are most mystics vegetarians to one degree or another and why do they fast?

Fasting sharpens and opens up the mind, heightens consciousness and eventually leads to a privileged relationship with the universe or a divine being. Even anorexics, who suffer from a serious eating disorder, are elated to feel lighter, more open, more intelligent and more quick-minded. Many are young girls who are ethereal in nature and excellent students.

Total fasting is obviously dangerous and must be prohibited, as it results in severe muscular loss and a deterioration of vital functions.

The protein diet resembles fasting in many ways: you eat less, much less even, but only for a limited period of time. Patients who go on a protein fast quickly realize after a few days that they are no longer hungry and that they have lost their food cravings. They can go into a pastry shop or look at a mouth-watering dish and not be the least bit tempted. All say they are more alert, keener, not fatigued and more energetic and that they are able to handle life's ups and downs better.

The protein diet induces *ketosis*, which makes your body produce amphetamine-like "ketonic bodies". Ketonic bodies are natural appetite suppressants, stimulate and sharpen the mind, and increase stamina. This is a win-win situation: you lose weight and feel great…

Hunger strikers know that they will eventually no longer feel the effects of a lack of food due to the amphetamine-like or appetite-suppressing effect of *ketosis*.

What Happens During *Ketosis*?

When you follow the protein diet, your pancreas rests because there is no sugar for it to detect. As a result, it no longer secretes insulin (only a small amount of insulin is produced for vital functions). Consequently, the over-heated furnace cools down and resets.

As long as the body is producing virtually no insulin, it is in a state of *ketosis*. It burns fat (and protein, if protein intake is inadequate) because it has no glucose for fuel.

- ***Ketosis* is a physiological phenomenon. There is no active slimming ingredient; however, a natural, physiological slimming response is triggered in the body.**

The body, deprived of carbohydrates, will first burn its glucose reserves in the liver and muscles. That takes about twelve hours. As a matter of fact, that's what happens every night — the period of the day when you go without food the longest and use up all of your available carbohydrates.

Let's suppose that your body has depleted its readily accessible carbohydrates and that it must burn fat to meet its energy needs. Luckily, there is a huge, almost unlimited supply of fat in theory.

All you have to do is trigger the burning of those reserves.

Any system that requires energy never uses up its reserves as long as it has fuel.

The very purpose of fat is to store energy.

Let's Talk Money

Your body manages its energy like you manage your finances (well, not too much we hope!). If you have a current account and a savings account, you won't have to dip into your savings account as long as your current account remains in the black. Your pocket book would have to be hopelessly empty before you would tap your savings,

Sugar is your current account when it comes to energy for living. As long as your body has sugar, it will not burn fat (it'll even accumulate fat if your insulin goes out of whack). When and only when it has no more sugar will your body begin to burn fat to meet its daily energy requirements.

When you lose weight, you live off your reserves.

That's why you must not eat any carbohydrates during the protein diet. Carbohydrates do not make you gain weight, but at this point in the process they'll keep you from losing weight, because they prevent the body from dipping into its reserves. As long as it has sugar, your body will not use its "fat savings".

- **Eliminate all slow and fast sugars from your diet so that you can live off your reserves.**

Living off the Right Reserves (off the wrong ones, actually)

The body has two types of reserves:

- lipids (fat); and

- protein (muscles and organs).

Fat loss is good; muscle loss is dangerous. Therefore, the diet – or the fast, if you prefer – must be supplemented with proteins to prevent muscle loss after your muscles have depleted their reserves and to encourage muscle-building as the diet goes along.

A major benefit is now clear: unlike other low-calorie diets, the protein diet does not reduce energy levels and many dieters experience increased energy levels.

If the body is deprived of sugar, where will it get its glucose?

A sedentary man who weighs 155 pounds has 33 pounds of useable fats (or 105,000 kilocalories), 13 pounds of useable protein in his muscles (or 25,000 kilocalories) and 6.5 ounces of glycogen in his liver and muscles (or 760 kilocalories).

After the body has depleted its reserve of carbohydrates, it is faced with an emergency: it must immediately find glucose in order to keep its vital organs functioning (the brain, heart, kidneys and red blood cells all need glucose).

Once its glycogen reserves have been depleted, the body begins to convert the amino acids found in muscle protein into glucose. This process – called gluconeogenesis – provides the body with precious glucose to replace the rapidly depleted glycogen reserves.

Glucose, however, is not the only useable fuel. The body also derives energy from its immense reserve of fatty tissue (fat cells). Fatty acids obtained from triglycerides in fat cells can be used by muscles, but not by the brain. Therefore, the body converts most of its fatty acids into substances called "ketonic bodies", which can be used by the brain. Ketonic bodies are a more refined fuel than fatty acids.

Ketosis is a biochemical process that allows the body to use fat as its main source of energy during a prolonged fast, while partially preventing muscle loss.

After the body has depleted its reserve of carbohydrates during a prolonged fast, it turns to fats and proteins. Fats are exactly what you want to burn in order to lose weight. Muscles, or proteins, on the other hand, are what you want to preserve at all cost.

Since the breakdown of fat is insufficient, your body also uses its other possible source of glucose: muscles. That's why a poorly designed diet results in fat and muscle loss. The body looks for energy, irrespective of whether that energy comes from fat or muscles, and must be given the necessary amount of proteins to prevent muscle loss.

8 The Protein Diet, Tried and True

Putting the body into a state of *ketosis* to force it to burn fat is nothing revolutionary. Blackburn, who pioneered the protein diet, introduced it in the United States in the 1970s and met with some success.

The Setbacks of the Blackburn Diet

Blackburn – like everyone else – started with the idea that you had to eat less to lose weight. The less you ate, the faster you lost weight. Of course, such fasting had a serious drawback: muscle loss. Since the heart is a muscle, heart attacks were also a concern.

Blackburn's theory was simple and focused on two principles:

- eat as little as possible, by developing a very low-calorie diet in order to create a negative caloric balance; and

- provide muscles and vital organs with an essential amount of proteins to ensure a nitrogenous balance.

To ensure rapid, healthy weight loss, Blackburn developed diets whose severe calorie restrictions were compensated by proteins, vitamins and mineral salts in proportion to the needs of male dieters (1.4 g of protein per kilogram of body weight) and female dieters (1.2 g of protein per kilogram of body weight).

This spawned two types of protein diets: one based on lean meat and fish and another based on powdered proteins obtained from animal sources (milk, collagen and gelatin) supplemented with mineral salts and mixed with water.

Americans were enthusiastic about Blackburn's hugely successful protein diet, but lacked objectivity and care. Protein packets were sold everywhere, and dieters thought they could dispense with the advice of nutritionists. Unwise dieters stuck with the diet for several weeks or months without the slightest supervision of a nutritionist.

A few consecutive protein diet incidents in 1977 sent shockwaves throughout the weight-loss community. Most involved cardiac patients who had gone on the diet without supervision and unfortunately paid the price. However, some victims had no heart trouble prior to going on the diet.

The proteins given to dieters were primarily obtained from hydrolyzed collagen or gelatin, two proteins that are low in essential amino acids, particularly in tryptophan, which is a precursor to serotonin – an anti-stress agent *par excellence*. (Of the 24 amino acids, the body makes 15. The other nine are essential amino acids that must be supplied by the diet.)

Everyone is well aware of how important serotonin, a neurotransmitter, is for the central nervous system. Most new-generation antidepressants like Prozac and Seropram are serotonergic.

After the above-mentioned disturbing incidents, dieters dropped the protein diets developed by Blackburn as quickly as they had adopted them, opting instead for new developments in dietetics without questioning the nature of the proteins the victims had eaten.

Let's not forget that all of this happened in the 1970s. At the time, research into the value of proteins, the body's real protein needs and the concept of biological value was still rather embryonic. The protein diet's bad reputation was here to stay given the depression, heart attacks and malnutrition it had caused.

Obviously, research has made progress and we now have a better understanding of the value of proteins, protein needs and biological value. In the end, Blackburn was right. However, the quality of the protein needed to be re-examined and a more stringent protocol including monitoring by a nutritionist was required.

Recent work has made it possible to identify the exact composition of an ideal protein based on such criteria as the chemical score, the digestive utilization coefficient (DUC), the Protein Digestibility Corrected Amino Acid Score (PDCAAS), and biological value. As well, indications and contraindications are thoroughly understood.

Animal or Vegetable?

Where do proteins come from? The answer is obvious: from animals (meat, fish, eggs, dairy products) and plants (grains and legumes).

Plant products that contain proteins can be preserved or dried. That's easy to remember.

Potatoes, a starchy food, cannot be dried because they contain no protein. Neither can lettuce, green beans, broccoli and all other green vegetables. No proteins, no dehydration.

Grains and pulses – think dried peas, chickpeas, field beans and lentils – can easily be preserved after they have been dehydrated.

It is generally accepted that animal proteins are superior to plant proteins because they are rich in essential amino acids. So how can we live without animal proteins? Large numbers of people do, because half the world's population is vegetarian. These people may have deficiencies, but they live rather healthy lives. And although there are millions of strict vegetarians by conviction or by force of circumstances, there are no strict carnivores (even the Inuit scoff down vegetables every chance they get). When babies are weaned, they are first fed baby cereal, fruit, vegetables, biscuits and bread crust, not meat.

Humans can live on plant proteins, provided they combine them (grain + legume).

Although they are extremely important, plant proteins are underrated. Combining plant proteins leads to a high-quality protein combination: legumes are rich in lysine, an essential amino acid, but poor in methionine, while grains are rich in methionine but low in lysine.

Many basic recipes used by impoverished people around the world combined grains and legumes: couscous was originally a dish of semolina and chickpeas. Indians in the Andes combined maize with red kidney beans. Even in France, cassoulet could be eaten without meat, provided the beans were covered with a layer of breadcrumbs. In Asia, there are rice and bean, rice and pea, rice and algae, and rice and mushroom recipes, which also contain proteins. Notice that all of these plant products can be dried.

The plant world still contains unknown riches like quinoa, a highly nutritional grain that is eaten in South America but virtually unheard of in Europe.

Why do most diets always recommend salads, broiled meat, fish, hard-boiled eggs and fat-free cottage cheese? Apart from the salads, these diets are almost exclusively based on animal protein for two reasons:

- We live in a carnivorous society which claims that meat is muscle and that when you eat meat, you build muscle. This is reasoning by similarity: you don't strengthen your heart by eating heart and you don't become less bald by eating hair.

- Grains and pulses contain plant proteins as well as a large amount of slow sugars or complex carbo-hydrates…

Is There an Ideal Protein?

What proteins are most likely to meet man's physiological needs? Complete proteins, ideally composed of amino acids and containing no fat or sugar, would, but they have no reason to exist. Your diet must include a wide variety of foods to ensure that your body has all the nutrients it needs: proteins, fats and sugars, as well as vitamins, trace elements and mineral salts. If a complete protein existed, it would decrease rather than increase the nutritional value of your diet.

A complete protein can be made from plant products (soya, which is a legume) and milk or eggs. The proteins in the protein diet are preparations that contain only the necessary protein elements. These substitute proteins are a major plus, because they combine the best elements of several substrates and can be enriched with as many vitamins, mineral salts and trace elements as needed.

9 The Protein Diet Phases

By now, you probably realize that overweight is a complex problem involving countless parameters. But you still haven't learned how to lose weight. What solution makes it possible to shed fat quickly while retaining muscle mass?

Consulting a Nutritionist

I gave you this lengthy history, because I give it to my patients.

I've found that your chances of following a treatment are better if you understand how you put on weight, how you can lose it, how your body stores and burns fat, what *ketosis* is and how it works. It's good to be familiar not only with the principles of dietetics, which are just now becoming widely known, but also with scientific concepts (anatomy, physiology, etc.) so that you will be less prone to overindulgence, backsliding, slips and frustration.

When patients see a nutritionist, they do not expect to be given a speech. They think the nutritionist will "weigh and measure them", assess the seriousness of their case on the BMI chart, conduct a brief dietary survey and, if necessary, ask them in a haughty tone to pinpoint their excesses or errors. Patients think the nutritionist will dwell on calorie charts and exclaim: "My, my, you're overeating!", or "Oh dear, you're not eating properly!" or "My goodness, your diet is awful!" Then patients expect the nutritionist to readjust and correct their diet after counting the calories and they hope to lose the extra pounds and keep them off.

If there is one constant in all of this (weights and measurements, questionnaire, dietary survey), it's that patients just cannot be expected to follow instructions and orders passively. They need to understand that they must take ownership of their weight loss. Weight loss is not owed to them and it does not occur without effort. Losing weight goes against nature and requires real motivation and vigilance.

The Protein Diet for Visible Weight Loss

In a nutshell, to lose weight you must go on a protein diet so that your pancreas can rest and *ketosis* can be induced in order to make your body burn fat. That implies eliminating sugars and protecting muscles by consuming an adequate amount of protein.

There are obviously nuances based on each dieter's physiology and the total number of pounds to be lost. In general, a woman who follows the protein diet for 20 days will lose eight to ten pounds, while a man will lose a little more.

The protein diet involves eating an exact amount of specific proteins.

Since there is no ideal protein, "ideal" meaning a pure (no fats and carbohydrates) and complete protein containing all essential amino acids, the solution is to use an ideally reconstituted protein. That's why the protein diet is based on protein powder substitutes that are mixed with water.

Why a Protein Substitute?

Everyday foods such as sugar, fruit and potatoes contain a host of pure carbohydrates. There are also pure fats like butter and olive oil. A word of caution though: purity should not be confused with natural. Butter and olive oil are not natural foods; they must be extracted or made from another food, but they are pure. The final product contains only fats.

As mentioned previously, since proteins do not occur in an isolated state, protein substitutes, or the missing link in our diet if you will, must be used. But the use of these proteins is not an end in itself. The goal is to remove them as other foods are progressively reintroduced.

Easy as 1-2-3

The protein diet is very simple: your nutritionist determines the number of protein packets you'll need each day. As a rule, you'll need three or four: one for breakfast, one for lunch and one for a late afternoon snack.

Some nutritionists suggest that you replace each meal with a protein packet. This is often unnecessary, as patients may become bored more quickly. One very low-calorie, carbo-hydrate-free meal per day will not compromise the method's efficacy and will keep boredom at bay. Again, the goal is to follow a protein diet that provides enough protein to protect your muscle mass, the heart included, rather than a high-protein diet. Again, your nutritionist will determine the optmum proportion of protein for you based on your individual situation, so that you'll lose fat and no muscle. Each case is unique.

At home, you'll need only dilute the contents of the packets in hot or cold water and cook or heat the mixture if necessary.

There's a wide range of flavours and textures so you won't get bored. You can enhance the mixes, provided you avoid products that will stall the weight loss (see the recipes in the appendices).

There is a wide range of mixes for vegetable, mushroom, tomato, chicken and fish soup; soufflés and omelettes; vegetable purees; classic puddings (vanilla, chocolate and butterscotch); fruit mousses and hot and cold drinks.

In addition to the required packets, you'll be able to eat an unlimited amount of most vegetables that you can prepare any way you like, provided you add no fat. Cook them en papillote or in a court bouillon, or steam them. Use all the seasoning, spices and herbs you want. They're recommended! You'll be given easy-to-prepare, delicious recipes so that you won't have the impression you're on a diet.

Eat Your Veggies!

All very low-glycemic index vegetables, or almost all vegetables, are allowed on the protein diet:

> • **Vegetables to Enjoy: asparagus, Swiss chard, celery, chicory, Chinese cabbage, cucumber, zucchini, watercress, endive, spinach, fennel, lettuce, mache (lamb's lettuce), sorrel, bell peppers, radishes.**

Other vegetables contain slightly more carbohydrates, but are still allowed (some nutritionists disallow them; however, if you don't overdo it, these vegetables will not keep you from losing weight).

- **Vegetables to Enjoy in Moderation: eggplant, broccoli, fresh button mushrooms, cabbage, sauerkraut, cauliflower, red cabbage, green beans, turnips, dandelion, leeks, soy sprouts, tomatoes.**

You'll have to give up the following vegetables temporarily:

- **Vegetables to Avoid: artichokes, beets, carrots, celeriac, Brussels sprouts, salsify.**

In general, a strict diet means a diet consisting solely of protein packets (4 to 5 per day) and green vegetables. I always allow one normal, light, carbohydrate-free meal. In fact, one-half pound of fish with green vegetables will not radically alter the diet, because one-quarter pound of white fish contains less than 2 grams of fat. And it allows you to keep up your social and family life. Paradoxically, the more weight you have to lose, the more this benefit is important.

So, do away with the protein packets at night and have a normal dinner with your family or friends. You'll be better off because of the social interaction. You can prepare a lean fish filet or cut of meat (turkey, chicken, guinea fowl, veal) accompanied by as many vegetables as you like, or you can prepare a protein packet.

What beverages may you drink while you're on the protein diet? Water and infusions (tea, coffee, herbal teas) without sugar or sweetened with aspartame. Drink plenty of fluids – Badoit or Vichy bottled mineral water, if possible – to prevent a sodium deficiency. (You consume less salt on the protein diet than you would when eating regular meals.) Some nutritionists recommend salt tablets (sodium chloride).

You'll be eating nothing else. Do not reduce the amounts determined for you, as that may be harmful to your health.

In summary, the foods you eat during the protein diet – the protein packets recommended by your nutritionist and all the raw or cooked vegetables you want – will put your body in a state of *ketosis*. You'll also be given vitamin, trace element and mineral salt supplements, because the protein diet does not provide your body with enough sodium, potassium, calcium or magnesium.

No Backsliding!

Eating the slightest amount of fast or slow sugars during the protein diet may stall weight loss for two to three days.

Don't go off track by eating a juicy hamburger, a slice of bread and butter or a fruit. Unfortunately, there is virtually no correlation between the seriousness of a slip and the weight-loss process. You may say to yourself that it's just once… you won't gain any weight… it's okay.

A slip won't make you gain weight, but it'll stall the weight-loss process. Why?

Weight loss is triggered when you eliminate carbohydrates from your diet. However, your body takes time to start burning fat after you've stopped eating carbohydrates. In other words, weight loss is not instantaneous.

The delay is how long it takes for a series of complex biochemical reactions to occur in the body. Even the slightest amount of sugar will put you back at square one, and you'll have to wait two to three days to start losing weight again, because that's how long the mechanism will take to get going.

If your nutritionist puts you on a strict, 20-day diet, you're on a diet for 20 consecutive days and not 20 days with breaks.

Backsliding may cause bouts of fatigue. In fact, as long as the body has no sugar, it produces no insulin and there's no hypoglycemia. When you eat sugar, you trigger the production of insulin and might become hypoglycemic and find yourself running out of steam, feeling light-headed, etc.

The Issue: Resurfacing after Total Immersion

The protein diet takes place over a limited period of time. If it helps, count the protein diet days you have left. It's not a lengthy diet like those frustrating, intolerable and seemingly endless low-calorie diets that cause much backsliding and failure (because they have no stabilization phase...).

The protein diet is not about dietetics or health practices; it's a diet or a therapeutic process. It's a treatment. You'll go back to eating a balanced diet afterwards.

- **A diet has a definite beginning and end: the concept of a time limit is very important.**

A diet is like deep-sea diving: a diver descends in one go with confidence because he knows he'll resurface. A diver always resurfaces in stages instead of in a single ascent, to allow his body to adapt to the change in pressure. He ascends in order to reach the surface and not to stay at a certain stage for the rest of his life, even if he's just 20 inches from the open air.

The purpose of a diet is to lose weight and then to stabilize it with a normal, balanced diet and not by eating three peas, two green beans and fat-free cottage cheese.

The protein diet has two goals:

- bring about rapid weight loss; and

- stabilize your new weight.

Keep in mind that these are two distinct "contracts" with different goals, methods and durations. Stabilization is not owed; it must be earned.

The fact that you successfully lost weight does not necessarily mean that you'll be able to stabilize your new weight over the long term. Oftentimes, patients think that eating normally is eating like they did before they went on the diet. The same causes produce the same effects: these patients might put back on the pounds because they revert to their old eating habits. That's normal and understandable, given our physiology.

The Intermediate Phases

After you've shed the extra pounds, you may gradually go back to eating normally prior to the stabilization phase. Think about that deep-sea diver coming up from a deep dive who needs decompression stops.

In your case, the "stops" involve gradually reintroducing normal foods to your diet that contain increasingly more calories, fats or carbohydrates, to ensure a smooth transition from the protein diet phase to the stabilization phase and so that your body can gradually become accustomed to these new additions.

What exactly do the intermediate stages involve? After the strict phase during which you eat three to four protein packets per day, one meal is reintroduced, followed by another and then breakfast and, finally, complex carbohydrates. There may be slight variations, because I recommend one light meal per day from the outset.

During Phase 2, the noon-hour packet is replaced with a meal similar to the one you have in the evening: white meat or fish, unlimited vegetables, a dairy product (low-fat cottage cheese or yogurt), with or without artificial sweetener.

No carbohydrates are added during this phase if you still need to lose some weight, so that *ketosis* is not interrupted.

Breakfast becomes more interesting during Phase 3 (yogurt, whole-wheat bread, cereal, etc.).

The phases vary from one individual to another, and each nutritionist adapts the protocol to each patient.

Step by step, a balanced diet is created with normal foods and the protein packets are phased out. Go by your nutritionist's advice, rather than by the instructions on the protein packets. Besides, the best protein firms never suggest a protocol since it varies from one individual to another.

The number of phases between the protein diet and the balanced maintenance phase depends on your nutritionist. In general, there are four phases:

- Phase 1: The protein diet, with three protein packets per day, and green vegetables;

- Phase 2: The lunch or dinner protein packet is replaced with your choice of 150 to 200 g of white meat or fish, along with green vegetables;

- Phase 3: Grains are gradually added to breakfast. Lunch and dinner still consist of lean meat or fish and green vegetables, plus a dairy product once every two days.

- Phase 4: This is the stabilization phase, which is a balanced maintenance diet (*cf.* Chapter 10).

The length of each phase varies and obviously depends on the total number of pounds to be lost.

In general, Phase 1 lasts as long as it takes to lose 70 to 80% of the total amount of weight to be lost. The remaining 20 to 30% of the weight is lost during the subsequent phases, although each case is unique.

Obviously, the phases for a person who needs to lose 8 to 10 pounds will not be the same as the phases for someone who needs to lose 80 to 100 pounds. In the latter case, the phases will be much longer. Your nutritionist will prepare a personalized schedule for you.

Supervision is Essential

Now that you have the protocol, do not go on an unsupervised diet. You must be supervised by a nutritionist who will look for any contraindications (*cf.* Chapter 17) and give you the mandatory vitamin, mineral salt and trace element supplements.

10 Stabilization

Change the way you think about food. After you've lost a few pounds on the protein diet phase (active weight loss), you'll quite rightly aspire to two things:

- stabilize your weight;

- enhance your food selection.

A Major Concern

Those who have lost weight are obviously concerned about stabilizing their weight, especially if they've experienced disheartening yo-yo weight loss and gain.

In my fifteen years of practice, my patients have always said: "I want to lose weight and keep it off."

The purpose of a diet is not only to bring about weight loss, but also to maintain the new weight. Stabilization is not difficult if it is considered work rather than something that is owed or a given. You must be keenly aware of your eating habits during the stabilization phase, and that's where dietetics comes in.

During a discussion on nutrition, a colleague remarked: "You always put the weight back on after you've completed the protein diet." So I handed him a piece of paper and asked him to write a protocol that would stop the pounds from coming back on. I said, after a long period of silence: "Dear colleague, haven't you confused weight loss with dietetics?"

During another conference, another colleague asked me: "What proves that the weight loss is permanent?"

"Well, nothing, my dear colleague, unless I eat for you", I replied.

You see, even doctors sometimes confuse a diet with dietetics.

- **Do not confuse weight loss with weight maintenance, or diet with weight stabilization. Both are two distinct processes and contracts.**

Some weight-loss diets are better than others, but generally speaking all diets result in weight loss.

If you want to stay at your ideal weight, you must go on a good diet and then focus on stabilizing your weight.

The purpose of a diet is to bring about weight loss. That's why it must not be a balanced diet (see Chapter 7). But you can't forever disregard the rules of dietetics that make it possible to maintain a desired weight if it's appropriate.

If a fire broke out in your house, you'd have the firefighters extinguish it. That's their job and they fulfill their contract. But if you asked them: "Since you're here, why don't you build me a new house and give me some fire-prevention tips?" they'd reply: "We can't do that; it's not our job. It's different work that requires a new contract."

That's exactly what happens with weight loss: you go on a diet to lose weight and the diet fulfills its mission. Maintaining your new, ideal weight is another job that requires a different contract and a different procedure.

This is No Food Free-for-All

The protein diet is followed by a stabilization phase. Then what? Are you finished? Are your worries over? Of course not. If you revert to overeating, you'll regain the weight you lost, albeit not as fast as with other diets.

Since nature programmed your body to store fat, you often gain four pounds or so in the fall in preparation for the winter. Or you gain weight after your holidays. Don't be alarmed. All you have to do is go back on the protein diet for ten days once a year. If you fail to take action, those four pounds a year will start to add up after a few years… Again, you must be careful. This is where dietetics comes in, as it teaches you the fundamentals of healthy eating. But that's for a later chapter.

Stabilization? What's That?

Stabilization is not a state (which is static by definition); it's a process, a job that requires effort. Here's another example: you're sitting in front of a speaker. You seem to do nothing but listen to him or her. However, you're actually trying to sit up straight and avoid slouching. Although you hardly realize it, you are making an effort.

During the stabilization phase, you'll be required to make such seemingly unnoticeable efforts as soon as you've understood the principle. You'll spontaneously put yourself back on track as soon as you catch yourself slacking off on the principles of dietetics.

Is this difficult and restricting? Not necessarily. If I give you a difficult job to do, you may not succeed despite your best efforts. But if you don't go out of your way to finish the job, you won't be able to say that the job was difficult because you never made a true effort. The same is true when you want to maintain your weight after you've been on a diet. Don't say it's difficult before you've even started. Motivation is the key.

Your Reward: A New Body

If you have a great deal of weight to lose, you want get out of your awkward, inelegant, uncomfortable body. You only see all those excess pounds and your personality has taken a back seat to your body, which literally and figuratively takes up a lot of space.

Having a body that does not match your true aspirations is like living in an apartment in a depressing and run-down neighbourhood that you just can't wait to leave.

Imagine living in a dilapidated apartment in a seedy part of town. The tagged staircase, the garbage in the elevator, the green spaces covered in dog waste and the vandalized mail boxes will eventually go unnoticed. Are you going to scrub the walls, repair the mailboxes, and hunt down the polluters? No, the situation has deteriorated to the point that you no longer care about your surroundings. You just can't be bothered, because this is not your home.

Once you're in your slim, toned-up body, you feel like a new person and rediscover your body. It's like returning to your home and maintaining it meticulously.

Once you've taken back the body you've always wanted, you won't let it deteriorate ever again. You will be able to stabilize your weight better because you will have set a goal for yourself. If a 220-pound person gains ten pounds, she won't notice. Her body is not her own. She lets the weight sneak up on her. After all, it doesn't really matter if she weights 220, 240 or 260 pounds.

As she drops the pounds, she'll become in harmony with her body and her body image, and she'll be more motivated by the visible results. Patients who succeed in losing a great deal of weight are pleasantly surprised by their reflection in shop windows. They feel like they're back in the real world of pleasures. They are outsiders no more.

These very same patients go on the offensive as soon as they gain three or four pounds and immediately do what it takes to keep their figure, because they had such a hard time attaining their ideal weight and don't want to fall back in the same trap. It's all about motivation.

Nip Apathy in the Bud

Disheartened patients try to shorten the intermediate phases just because they're fed up.

They discontinue the protein diet because they find it too difficult, attempt to stabilize their weight on their own, and plan to go back on the diet as soon as they have more willpower. That attitude leads to failure.

Each patient determined the weight they wanted to attain along with the help of their nutritionist. The patient and the nutritionist signed a moral contract and as long as the target weight has not been reached, their work isn't finished and unfinished work has no value. They don't have the courage to go on and they're in a temporary, precarious situation. Precariousness leads to weight gain instead of weight loss.

If I build a sandcastle on the beach with some children and it never gets past the first stage, I won't be upset if it's washed away by the ocean or destroyed by passers-by. But if I create a magnificent sandcastle that's swept away by a wave, I will be heartbroken.

That's why it's important to finish the job, fulfill the contract and reach your goal with unflinching determination. Once you've attained your ideal weight, you'll have to watch your weight closely.

Restoring Balance

Your aim is to go back to eating a balanced diet. And that's good. But what is a balanced diet?

Nowadays, people unfortunately tend to think that a balanced meal is a full meal that includes a little bit of everything: appetizers, meat or fish, vegetables, bread, cheese, and fruit or a dessert. So you've got crudités, animal protein, dairy products, grains, and slow and fast carbohydrates.

According to widely accepted, conventional dietetics, a balanced diet means eating a reasonable amount of everything at each meal.

So it's only natural to think that a balanced diet must be modeled on a full meal. We all know of mothers who often worry if their children are eating a complete meal – or a balanced one in their minds – at the school cafeteria.

I have a slightly different view of what a balanced diet is and suggest that you change your way of thinking. A diet must be balanced throughout the day and not at each meal.

You'll be fine if you eat the foods your body needs in a 24-hour period. It'll lack nothing and you won't experience any nutritional deficiencies, health problems or weight gain.

A full meal is nothing more than a meal that's difficult... to digest. Bread, meat, beans, fruit, cheese, fish and vegetables are not all digested in the same way. Besides, we never ate full meals in the past.

The mantra for the stabilization phase is dissociation.

Let me explain: the dissociated diet is primarily for individuals who are in the stabilization phase or overweight. Everything is dictated by metabolism, although some individuals do not need to separate foods due to a fluke of genetics. The principle of dissociation that I advocate is not a principle of general dietetics or healthy eating practices. It's for people who have a tendency to gain weight.

Dissociation is the Key

You're surprised again: you know that dissociated diets have recently wreaked havoc and you can't see yourself eating only carbohydrates one day and fats or proteins the next. And you shudder at the thought of eating only beans one day, cheese the next day and brown rice the day after that.

That's not what a dissociated diet is at all. Let's recap: the objective is to balance all food groups during a day so that you eat a little of everything over a 24-hour period. No deficiencies, no boredom. You may eat a little of everything, but not at one meal.

Carbohydrates and fats cause weight gain? Solution: separate them, like a teacher separates two troublesome students.

Dissociation is nothing new. Initially, dissociation was nothing less than culinary cruelty: meat on Monday, dairy products on Tuesday, fruit on Wednesday, and so on. Then the nutritionist Shelton proposed a less systematic and more user-friendly daily approach: dairy products for breakfast, animal proteins for lunch and vegetables for dinner, and a total ban on simple and complex carbohydrates. His method results in rapid weight loss primarily because you eat less. Boredom, restrictions and frustration lurk; your social life suffers the consequences and there's no more joy in eating. Soon you've had enough and give up.

Not all foods can be dissociated all the time, because that would create deficiencies. Plus, dissociation is impractical and leads to boredom, which is sure to result in the diet being stopped. You don't live in a bubble and usually eat at your workplace restaurant, at a neighbourhood café, at friends' homes, on the go… Complete separation of foods is enormously complicated when it comes to managing and preparing meals.

The stabilization meal I propose is not restrictive. With a little bit of care, you'll be able to eat your meals anywhere, whatever the circumstances: at home or at work, at a self-service restaurant or at a local café that has a daily special.

11 An Easy Maintenance Diet

During the maintenance phase, you'll eat a full and varied diet that includes carbohydrates and fats (in moderation, of course), which are separated during the day: no carbohydrates at noon and no fats in the evening.

Breakfast

Think of your standard continental breakfast with carbo-hydrates and proteins (a little):

- Whole-wheat bread or cereal. The bread may be lightly buttered or spread with a thin layer of light jam.

- A dairy product: yogurt or cottage cheese, or a hard cheese from time to time.

- A fruit or fruit juice, if you wish.

- A hot drink: tea or coffee (unsweetened or sweetened with an artificial sweetener).

Ideally, an English breakfast is better because of its proteins (eggs, bacon or ham, cheese). The proteins, acting in tandem with the carbohydrates, are better at controlling the threat of hypoglycemia, because they lower the breakfast's total glycemic index. So go ahead and have an English breakfast if you prefer.

You have no doubt put your finger on an aberration: buttered bread. What happened to the principle of dissociation? Why are the carbohydrates in the bread combined with the fats in the butter? To make an exception for the continental breakfast and avoid breaking with tradition. Be sure to use a knob of butter and not half a pound!

Lunch

Lunch is often eaten outside the home. Since most workplace restaurants allow you to choose your dishes, you'll be able to follow your stabilization diet.

- You can eat crudités if you wish, although they're not mandatory.

- Basic meal: meat or fish, preferably lean meat and no sauce.

- Side dish: vegetables; fats are tolerated because they can't be avoided. Besides, fats are virtually unavoidable in crudités, vegetables, meat and fish.

- A dairy product: cheese to accompany your salad, cottage cheese, yogurt.

Foods not permitted: simple or complex carbohydrates. You'll have to say good-dye to starchy foods, pasta, rice and potatoes. It's virtually impossible to find fat-free starchy foods unless you prepare them at home. Remember these figures: 100 grams of plain potatoes contains 80 calories, while the same amount of fries contains a whopping 400!

Bread is also banished, as are all sweet-tasting foods: fruit, dessert pastries and cream desserts.

In summary, lunch consists of a starter, a meat or fish dish with vegetables, and yogurt or cheese.

In the Afternoon

Some people still long for their childhood snacks, and we all sometimes get that empty feeling when the late afternoon rolls around.

Theoretically, after you've gone on the protein diet and lessened demands on your pancreas, you don't really need a snack because you won't be hypoglycemic on a regular basis. But if you want a snack, choose one of the following:

- a fruit;

- some yogurt;

- a whole-grain muffin with a small piece of dark chocolate.

Make the most of your afternoon snack. Chocolate is allowed because it won't make you gain weight.

Don't overdo it, though. Your afternoon snack is not supposed to look like a child's snack!

Dinner

Dinner is usually eaten at home. Most diets neglect, banish or shrink it. We've become accustomed to saying "eat breakfast like a king, lunch like a prince and dinner like a pauper".

That notion is outdated. Dinner has two roles:

- help you recover from your day and recharge your batteries;

- prepare for the next day.

Dinner is the last meal before the longest period that your body fasts: night-time.

For dinner, you'll have:

- 150 to 200 g complex carbohydrates, weighed and cooked. There are three kinds of complex carbohydrates:

  • starchy foods, like potatoes, which are not that great because they contain no protein and have a fairly high glycemic index;

  • grains: wheat, bulgur, buckwheat, corn;

  • pulses: lentils, field beans, chickpeas.

To summarize, you can choose from rice, pasta, lentils, semolina, green peas, beans, potatoes, wheat or buckwheat, as all contain complex carbs.

However, be moderate: one portion is 150 to 200 grams, and not three heaping servings under the pretext that it's allowed. Obviously, four-cheese pasta is much more fattening than pasta topped with tomato sauce.

The important thing to remember is that your dinner must contain little to no fat. Feel free to sprinkle some Parmesan cheese on your pasta, but don't use the entire package. You may also prepare a vegetable sauce using a smidgen of olive oil.

- You may have an unlimited amount of fresh vegetables

in addition to the complex carbohydrates.

- End your meal with a not-too-sweet dessert – homemade if possible – such as a semolina cake, rice pudding (you may have complex carbohydrates at night), a fruit or yogurt. Indulge in an evening dessert, because you never had one at lunchtime.

Your evening dinner need not include meat, fish or eggs, as you already had animal protein at lunchtime. Two servings of animal protein per day are too much. If you really can't do without protein, you may have a slice of ham, an egg or a fish filet for the sake of it.

In summary, your dinner consists of:

- complex carbohydrates;

- unlimited vegetables; and

- a dessert.

Be sure to limit the amount of white bread, which is considered a complex carbohydrate but acts like a simple carbohydrate. Cravings for white bread can be as strong as cravings for chocolate! (See the Glycemic Index in Appendix 2.)

As you read these recommendations for dinner, you're eyes are probably becoming as big as saucers. What you just read is not at all what you learned about the proper management of eating in the evening.

What? Starchy foods in the evening? Carbohydrates? You can feel your hips widen, because you do nothing but sleep at night. You find the idea shocking and think that starchy foods are heavy and difficult to digest. Are you that sure? Starchy foods are filling, that's for sure. But compare the damage done by eating 300 grams of pasta (carbohydrates), 300 grams of steak (proteins) or 300 grams of butter (fat), and you'll see that pasta is the easiest on your digestive system. We'll examine that in the next chapter.

The Evening Dinner Make-over

Why not eat your vegetables and starchy foods in a soup? Soup, a cornerstone of the European diet if not the global diet, particularly among the impoverished up until the mid-20th century, deserves a make-over.

Carbohydrates and vegetables are satisfying and filling. For starters, soup is hot and hot foods are more satisfying than cold foods.

In addition, you need to sit down to enjoy a bowl of soup, because it's hard to balance a hot bowl on your lap or eat soup while watching television. The rite in itself is calming and melts away stress. Without your being aware of it, you'll be taking the time to eat an evening dinner, which is not such a bad thing in today's fast-paced society. It's an opportunity to rediscover the joys of the family meal and to take stock of the day with your children.

They don't like soup? Perhaps you served it to them with some hesitation. There are all kinds of soups for all kinds of palates. All you need to do is find the right recipes.

Slow Down

Whether or not your menu includes soup, take the time to sit down comfortably at a table and enjoy your meal, even if you're dining solo. You'll gain more weight if you inhale your meal than if you take the time to enjoy it. The time it takes to digest food is inversely proportional to the length of your meal, because when food is properly chewed and adequately mixed with saliva, digestion is already underway.

12 Why Complex Carbohydrates in the Evening?

You must eat some carbohydrates in the evening to ensure the stabilization phase is a success. This requirement is invariably food for thought at this stage in the consultation. Here's the argument against eating carbohydrates in the evening: the carbs you eat in the evening are immediately stored by the body, because you sleep at night and don't burn them off through exercise.

Obviously, when patients tell me this, I ask them: "So when is the best time of day to eat carbohydrates?" They always reply that lunchtime is the best time. Why? "C'mon, doctor, because you can burn them off during the afternoon as you go about your business!"

That's a mistake and a sign that they aren't familiar with the digestive process.

What About Marathon Runners?

High-level athletes are usually under very close medical and dietetic supervision. Their problem is not losing weight, but rather retaining muscle mass and ensuring they are in the best shape possible for training and competition.

Have you ever asked a marathon runner how he prepares for 26-mile run? He wolfs down mountains of pasta, and that's not so he can go out and run all night. Similarly, the Tour de France has never taken place at night. Athletes, marathon runners and cyclists eat carbohydrates in the evening in order to build up reserves for the next day, when they'll have to perform at their best.

Do you see what I'm getting at? The digestion of simple and complex carbohydrates is one thing, and their release as a source of energy is another.

Let's go back to the example of the marathon runner. He eats pasta or other complex carbohydrates around 8 or 9 p.m. and sleeps like everyone else, digesting the carbohydrates he just ate and storing them in the form of glycogen in his liver and muscles. The next morning, he awakens full of energy and is ready for the marathon, because he'll be able to draw on the carbohydrate reserves his body made the night before.

You're an Athlete

You're not all that different from famous athletes. Your body functions in the same way as theirs. You need to build up your carbohydrates at night so that you can use them throughout the next day.

- **One important detail: complex carbohydrates have to be digested before they can be used.**

Digestion is the process by which food is broken up and converted into a substance suitable for absorption and assimilation into the body. Digestion is work, while burning reserves provides energy. And your body can only use the final product. As long as the work, or digestion, is incomplete, you have no reserves to burn.

You Don't Burn Energy in Real Time

A light needs electric current in order to light up a room. If you unplug it, it'll go out. Unlike the human body, it consumes energy in real time.

As you read these lines, you are probably not eating but your body is still functioning.

We use stored energy – our reserve of sugar or glycogen stored in the liver and muscles mostly during sleep, the recovery phase.

Remember that most of the time (when you're not eating), your body only uses carbohydrates for fuel rather than proteins or fats.

Sugar is the fuel of which you have the least and need the most. Since your body has no sugar cells, it's important that you regularly replenish your reserve.

If you eat only a little in the evening, like a slice of ham, a leaf of lettuce and some fat-free cottage cheese, as was recommended for many years, you'll feel fine the next morning because you'll still have a small reserve of glycogen. As the day goes by, you'll run out of sugar and might feel weak by late afternoon, because you've used up all your available reserves.

Imagine a long-range aircraft that stops to refuel and then continues its flight safely. Obviously, it could have continued flying for a while by running on its fumes. However, if it doesn't make a refuelling stop it'll run out of fuel above the ocean and won't be able to land safely at the airport of destination.

The comparison is self-explanatory. If you don't want to run out of energy by 6 p.m., you'll have to plan ahead and build up your supply of carbohydrates or fuel.

Would you fill your gas tank one litre at a time during a long road trip? Of course you wouldn't. You'd fill it up and hit the road with peace of mind.

The same applies to your glycogen reserves. After your body has digested and stored complex sugars, the replenished stock is ready for use and you won't run out of steam.

Your glycogen reserves must be replenished while you sleep for use the next day, just like an electric car whose battery is recharged overnight.

What if You Ate Some Carbs at Noon Anyway?

Do as you have been taught. Have some complex carbohydrates at noon; however, you won't be able to use them for energy for most of the afternoon because they won't be available. The amount of carbohydrates in the bloodstream that are ready for immediate use is negligible compared to what your body needs. Your body needs to be able to access its glycogen reserves, but has not had time to replenish them. So, your body takes all afternoon to digest those complex carbohydrates you had for lunch, which makes you feel somewhat drowsy because digestion burns calories, uses up energy and is tiring.

You'll still have a small amount of energy reserves the next morning, but as the day goes on you'll run out of steam and by 6 p.m. you'll have almost no energy reserves. Meanwhile, the complex carbs you had for lunch are not yet ready for use because they're still being digested.

The Other Alternative

Take my suggestion. Eat your complex carbohydrates in the evening, as do athletes, because you're a champion at everyday living. While you rest and sleep at night, your body will have time to replenish its energy reserve. Your digestive system does its work, calmly converting the nutrients (complex carbohydrates) you had for dinner into energy. The next morning, your supply of glycogen is ready for use throughout the day. At noon, you'll be able to get by with a carb-free lunch because any carbohydrates you do eat won't be converted into energy until the end of the day.

If you eat in this manner, you'll use up your energy reserves steadily. They won't needlessly fill up your fat cells and sugars won't be stored. This is a double dividend: you avoid hypoglycemic spikes and won't wolf down sweets.

The Dinner Revolution

When you eat complex carbohydrates in the evening, your body can build up its reserves and gradually retrain your pancreas. Dieters find this very disturbing: they have been told time and again that they must eat very little in the evening and limit pasta to twice a week. And now they're being told to eat carbohydrates in the evening, every evening as a matter of fact! What a revolution.

Dieters soon realize that they've changed their metabolism: their weight is stabilized and gone are the hunger pangs and postprandial drowsiness. They feel great all day long. All their friends are amazed. The diet works! It's all about logic and common sense. This diet approach is akin to the chrono-biological approach.

You're probably wondering how long you have to follow these recommendations. For the rest of your life? You'll have to follow them as long as possible after you've completed the diet. Your body feels good because you separate fats and carbohydrates and eat complex carbohydrates in the evening. A few months would be good. Frustrated? A few months is too long? No problem! You are entitled to go off the diet wagon once in a while…

13 Getting Back on Track

Once you've reached your ideal weight and are following the stabilization phase over the long term (rather long), you'll realize that you want the occasional "reward", the right to eat something that you fancy, something that is not forbidden. Or you'd like to have guests for dinner or be invited to dinner. In fact, you're a bit tired of precisely controlling what you eat. Don't panic; we'll teach you how to accommodate the inevitable slips.

Don't Give up Pleasure

It's simply unbearable to have to control what you eat for the rest of your life and deny yourself the dishes you love. We all like pleasure, and the pleasure of eating is one of life's greatest pleasures, especially in France which has a great reputation when it comes to enjoying fine food.

Some low-calorie diets suggest one thing and one thing only: endless no-no's. We're not about that at all: slips are not very serious as long as you know how to manage them.

Well, you say: "But how can I resist gourmandizing? If I let myself bend the rules ever so slightly, I'll be on a slippery slope and crave all the foods I love. I'd rather avoid temptation."

Be careful, you have mixed up two concepts: addiction and pleasure; the compulsion to wolf something down and hedonism.

Eating is essential and vital, much more essential than procreation. An ill-fed, malnourished woman does not menstruate. Her fertility – and that of an obese woman – is zero. You see, everything is linked.

Appreciate What's Good, It's Normal!

Try to distinguish pleasure from satisfaction. If you give me a box of chocolates, I'll enjoy one or two. But if I eat three or four and then polish off the box, that's not pleasure, that's satisfaction and I have satisfied only a need. Satisfy a need? Which one? That's the question.

Rarely are people totally deprived of their sense of taste. Those who cannot taste consider their handicap as unpleasant as mutilation or an amputation as they conceive it. Even those who claim they are not interested in the matter, like the fact that food is pleasing. You'd never eat something disgusting or that was ruined by oversalting, for example.

It's normal to appreciate a tasty dish or a healthy food.

Cravings are not normal. And more often than not, cravings are for sugar which can be considered a drug.

Some women say that they are "spontaneously"' attracted to carbohydrates. That's only partially true. Their pancreas is usually in overdrive, which leads them to think they need sugar. They always need more....

As soon as they go on the protein diet, they no longer consider the pleasure of eating sugar an irrepressible compulsion because the protein diet suppresses the appetite and retrains their pancreas.

They're able to enjoy a dessert without craving more; they're able to eat a piece of chocolate without eating the entire bar in one day; they have periodic, reasonable cravings that they are able to control; they no longer have a psychological need for sugar.

Neither patients nor nutritionists can ignore something as essential as the pleasure of eating. How many times have you heard of nutritionists who made their patients feel guilty? "You've fallen off your diet again, I'm sure you're cheating...." These investigators, who were numerous some twenty years ago, are on their way out because, according to psychology, it's better to convince than to antagonize and because yo-yoing is inevitable. Nevertheless, many dieters ended up feeling guilty as soon as they set their eyes on half a cookie, a drop of wine, a spoonful of sauce, or a slice of baguette. Their frustration was so intense that they eventually said: "What the heck, I'll go off the diet and eat whatever I want."

What's a Slip?

With the protein diet, you can eat what you like by managing the slips and without ruining the diet. The stabilization phase sets new rules: you may eat a little of everything and slip from time to time, provided you deal with the slips well.

Before looking at diet slips, let's talk about the path. Imagine you're driving aimlessly in the middle of the desert without a single point of reference or destination. You can swerve to the left and the right and weave through the sand without breaking a single traffic rule. On the freeway, however, you must drive in a more or less straight line and be acutely aware of your destination. The slightest turn of the wheel will make your vehicle leave the road. That's a diet detour or a swerve in the driving sense.

A diet detour occurs when you are aware that you are an active participant in your diet and the stabilization phase, which require you to show willpower and to be alert, motivated and steadfast just like when you're driving on the freeway. A slip is meaningless if there is no clear guideline.

Your stabilization phase is not exactly like driving on the freeway, because the slightest slip will be inconsequential if it is well managed.

You must first know what a slip is. If you allow your diet to go off course frequently, you will no longer be in the stabilization phase, you will have breached your contract, and your nutritionist will be unable to help you. One slip is a slip, while repeated slips are a bad habit.

Minor or Major Slip?

Once you realize that you are going off track or are about to – family celebration, restaurant invitation, office party – and have identified the danger, you must ask yourself one question: Am I setting myself up for a minor or a truly major slip? Each is dealt with differently.

A slip is minor if you watch what you eat, select your dishes and harmonize them as best possible with the rules of stabilization. Let's say that you have an hour to grab a bite to eat before going to a show. You go to a small restaurant and although you can't avoid fats, you can put your meal together wisely. Go for a starter and a main dish rather than a main dish and a dessert. Stay away from starchy foods, bread, pasta, fries, desserts, except maybe sugar-free yogurt. In so doing, you'll respect the rule of dissociation: do not combine carbohydrates and fats during one meal. You'll say: "Yes, but it's evening and I haven't had my portion of complex carbohydrates." You'll just have to skip them.

How do you make up for the slip? You don't. I don't think you slipped (you followed the rule of dissociation) and your well-trained body will eliminate the excess (fat and calories).

But isn't this type of slip minor in relation to other types of temptations, like a gala dinner, an invitation to a fine restaurant, or an evening with friends who have gone all out in your honour?

You don't want to disappoint the hostess or the person who invited you. Similarly, you enjoy a tasty raclette as much as anyone else in the winter. When at a wedding, you want to do justice to the delicious dishes and the tiered cake, celebrate along with everyone else and indulge.

On special occasions, throw out (only once!) the principles you have followed so closely. Go by the rules of friendship or society and forget about the rules of dietetics. Never mind the rule of food dissociation, eat what you fancy and spoil yourself for once.

Put yourself back on track after the excitement of the celebration has subsided.

The instructions are simple: the day after the event, avoid all simple and complex carbohydrates. Just for one day.

There is no need to make up for your excesses for an entire week or even for two or three days. One carb-free day will suffice.

The goal, as you well know, is not to lose weight (you already did that on the protein diet), but to make up for your diet detours, your one-day or one-meal overindulgence. The goal of the carb-free day is to prevent the fat from being stored in your fat cells.

Why? Your body needs sugar to be able to store fat in your fat cells. If you eat no sugar the day following the event, your pancreas will not produce any insulin and the fats you ate the night before will not be stored in your fat cells and will be eliminated instead. By avoiding all carbohydrates, you've stopped the process.

Just because you ate some fat, doesn't mean you'll immediately gain weight. Your body doesn't work that fast. If you eliminate all sugars the day after your diet slip-up, you'll have more or less undone the damage.

The stabilization phase is definitely much less restrictive than you feared, because it does allow some splurges. Just be sure to distinguish one-time slips from bad habits. You can't just alternate between days of feasting and days of no sugar. As with everything else, if you do not have a clear idea of your goal – maintaining your ideal weight – you'll likely fail.

Ideally, you'd go on the protein diet for one day after you've fallen off the diet wagon, but you don't always have those protein packets handy. Instead, have a coffee or tea and a yogurt for breakfast, and a small serving of lean meat or fish with green vegetables for lunch and dinner.

Besides, a dinner that puts you off track is often a copious dinner that lasts well beyond 8 p.m. You may not feel like eating a plentiful breakfast the next morning and be happy with a light lunch and dinner. That's enough to deal with a major diet slip-up.

14 They're All Against You

When you want to lose weight you sometimes get the feeling that there's a conspiracy to prevent you from succeeding.

You already know that your body is designed to store fat in order to prepare for any upcoming difficult periods and that it definitely is not designed to waste its reserves. It releases reserves sparingly, which makes dieting so difficult and so tricky psychologically. That's the biological reason, but it's not the only reason.

Blame Society

You have to be mentally strong to lose weight. You need willpower, there's no doubt about that. It would be dishonest to say that losing weight is easy and fun.

The protein diet allows you to shed those unwanted pounds with as little hassle as possible, and faster than other diets. Nevertheless, like any other diet, the protein diet deprives you of some foods that you love or love too much, such as anything fat or sweet. You often gain weight because you regularly eat fat or sweet foods. It's not necessarily your fault. It's because your pancreas is in overdrive or because you eat "comfort" foods to get through life's challenges.

We live in a difficult world in which many people are stressed, because job instability affects them one way or another or because they have numerous roles, responsibilities and obligations. And they always strive to do their best.

The Burden of Stress

There has been a steady drumbeat to end mediocrity. The bar is constantly being raised at work, in friendships and intimate relationships, in child rearing, and even in recreational activities. And then there's commuting, picking up the kids at daycare, taking them to the doctor or to a piano lesson, meeting professional and family obligations, the need to juggle schedules like finances are juggled. Life may well be easier in some respects, but it's mentally exhausting. Perfectionism is stressful… It may be a matter of survival, it may be due to feelings of guilt for those who do not assume, or have difficulty assuming their responsibilities or it may be about coping with what others think.

Way back when the human body needed every single calorie provided by food, stress made it possible to face difficult situations. The body had to build up its calorie stores to prepare for unforeseen situations requiring brief but intense energy use. The body had to be able to draw on its reserves quickly, as most situations were very physically demanding (hunting, outrunning the enemy, fighting, carrying game on one's back).

The human body's physiology has not changed radically over the last few hundreds of thousands of years. It understands all the warning signals very well: if there is stress on the horizon, it builds up reserves.

The problem is that nowadays, most stressful situations are not resolved physically. What's more, stress has gone from being an isolated event to something permanent and insidious. It affects your morale day in, day out.

The physiological system of stress, which supplies adrenaline and noradrenaline in milliseconds to cope with brief and intense stressful situations, is ineffective for long-term stress. An abnormal signal triggers an abnormal response in the body. A one-time stressful situation causes glycogen reserves to be used up and theoretically results in weight loss. A long-term stressful situation leads to weight gain in about half of the cases, because some people do lose weight during times of extreme stress. But that's not necessarily a good thing...

Each time you react to stress physically (giving your boss a piece of your mind, kicking something to vent off your anger), your body manages to overcome the need to let off steam by other means, like food.

The Burden of Conditioning

The above physiological factors are compounded by economic factors in Western nations.

We are constantly urged to eat more and more, and the fatter the food is, the better. Advertising, especially prime-time TV commercials, largely focus on sugar-containing products: beverages, desserts and cakes. Ads for deli meats and prepared meals abound – "rillette", ham, sausages, prepared dishes – all of which contain artery-clogging animal fat.

Worse yet, children, who lack the critical thinking skills needed to separate good foods from bad, are the prime target of this advertising.

Marketers can easily play on cravings, salivation and immediate desire. Obviously, these harmful practices make it harder to stay on a healthy diet and to educate children about nutrition.

Eating Disorders

All those commercials lead to abnormal eating habits that are affecting ever-larger proportions of children and young people.

Bulimia strikes early. An infant could live on milk, cereal, fruit and vegetables until at least the age of one. When meat and other animal proteins (with the exception of dairy products) are introduced early into a baby's diet, that baby will be predisposed to obesity.

Are you a couch potato? How long will it take for the high rates of youth obesity in the U.S.A. to be reached in France? The latest popular treatment for obese youth is an exercise bike generator that powers a television. If you don't want to miss a part of your television show, you must keep on pedaling. And don't even think about eating while you pedal, because the television will go off as soon as you remove a hand from the handlebars. More exercise and less snacking have reportedly yielded stellar results, because these children quickly went back to their normal, healthy figure. But at what cost, when they should be spending more time playing outside and less time in front of a screen, and when they should be happy with a muffin or a "plain" piece of chocolate rather than high-calorie, high-carb foods washed down with soda.

Anorexia, an eating disorder, mainly affects young girls who have berated themselves after a bulimic episode or just because they are a too plump. Anorexia is a serious eating disorder that is extremely difficult to treat and that absolutely requires the help of a specialist. Anorexics are proud of their diaphanous hands, bones that show through their skin and slender body. To them, eating is torture and they'll refuse to eat as long as they possibly can. Anorexia is dangerous and cause for immediate concern.

What About Your Family?

Life is stressful and we're constantly bombarded with advertising and incentives, and when you go on a protein diet you'll be under other kinds of pressure: your friends' benevolent doubt, family members' opinions and perhaps criticism ("why did you change your way of eating?") and critics. Defend yourself by using the solid arguments in favour of this method's results: rapid weight loss, improved morale as the pounds melt away, completely safe, healthier eating habits. Anyone who goes on the protein diet is better for it. Expect resistance, questions, doubt, and even warnings ("it's dangerous", "be careful"). Be strong and be sure of yourself. In this book you'll find all the proof you need that this weight-loss method is a physiological, natural and safe method.

As time goes by, your critics may start to support you. Eventually, they'll all want to use the method and you'll be giving them addresses and tips. What a pleasant turn of events – sceptics are following your lead!

Ignore Unsettling Remarks

Oftentimes, dieters who must contend with comments by friends and family are not on their first diet. They've decided to follow the protein diet because previous diets failed. Perhaps they've gone on so many unsuccessful diets that they've been weakened, ridiculed or the target of scepticism.

Here is a sampling of comments heard by patients.

Demotivating comments:

> "Don't waste your time with another diet. You'll just go off the diet anyway and regain all the weight you lost", or "I know someone who went on that diet and they put all the pounds back on".

Scepticism:

> "You think it'll work? After all, you have no reason to think you'll succeed based on all the other diets...."

Temptation:

> "Go on, have just a little; it's so good. A tiny serving won't ruin your diet and make you put back on some weight."

Attempts to throw you off track:

> "Well, well, you're not allowed to eat any fruit? That's odd. It's not very healthy either. Fruit is good for you; it's full of vitamins. It's not right to ban fruits, especially since they don't make you gain weight."

Attempts to make you worry or feel guilty:

> "I talked with so-and-so who went on the diet you're on and I read it in magazines: your diet is harmful to your health."

Obliging:

> "You should stop losing weight. You look fine the way you are."

It's hard to avoid comments that are allegedly made for "your own good". Don't let these hurtful people lead you to question your intentions. You decided to lose weight, and whatever happens is the result of a contract between you and your nutritionist. When you have faith in your nutritionist and their method, weight loss is a personal matter, so ignore these birds of ill omen.

Be a Survivor

It's hard to overhaul the eating habits you acquired during childhood.

Our relationship with food as a child is probably the only one that is carried over into adulthood. It's why eating disorders are often closely associated with emotions.

Unless you seek long-term counselling, you'll have a hard time ridding yourself of deeply instilled eating habits. You can try to distance yourself emotionally from food and adopt a more rational and less adversarial relationship with it. Whatever you do, an eating disorder is often a sign of internal emotional struggles stemming from an unsatisfying emotional life, conflicts in job duties, fear of becoming unemployed, difficult living conditions, or an unstable or insecure life.

If a person needs to lose 50 or 60 pounds, people consider them victim. Carrying all those extra pounds is like a curse. "Poor guy, he deserves to be pitied. Poor thing; it's a shame she has all that extra weight."

If such a person goes on a diet, they initially get all the support they need. However, human nature being what it is, we become suspicious of those who succeed.

Women who have lost a great deal of weight are often the prime target of animosity: others become jealous and sharp-tongued, saying that their gait and attitude have changed along with their figure.

If your legs are thinner, your thighs won't rub together anymore and you'll have an easier time walking. You'll feel more comfortable and at ease. Jealous men (and women) sense renewed rivalry, which leads them to make barbs for which you must prepare yourself.

Leaving jealousy aside, when you lose weight successfully you've completed a successful project. That success may contrast with the failures and dissatisfaction experienced by your friends and family members, and highlight their own difficulties.

Get Cooking!

Dieters have one final hurdle: cooking.

Make sure that you always have a good supply of protein diet packets so that you won't run out and stop *ketosis* and so that your body will be able to stock up on proteins every day.

Also, make sure that you have an ample supply of vegetables. Head to the supermarket and load up your cart with fresh vegetables (frozen vegetables are acceptable, too).

You'll find out that you need lots of vegetables because their volume decreases when cooked. Expect to spend more time in the kitchen, because vegetables take time to prepare: peeling, blanching, draining, subsequent preparation with spices, herbs and seasoning. Cooking vegetables involves many steps which may be new to you. Many young women who have lived off prepared meals are surprised at the recommendation that they cook. Cooking is a pleasure you're going to have to take up. Discover fresh herbs and spices, experience new food combinations. You'll see that it's fun and you won't have to eat plain vegetables, which may seem nice at the start of the protein diet (you'll have the impression that you're rediscovering true flavours), but which end up tasting bland or flavourless because they're unseasoned. You'll probably have many recipe ideas.

15 Exercise, the Finishing Touch

What do you really want to achieve by shedding all those pounds? Of course you want a thinner body. Do you want to measure up to the idealized body image? You know that won't suffice. You must also cut a fine figure.

Muscle Up

A pretty figure is more than a given weight or your height-to-weight ratio – your BMI. Sooner or later, you'll realize that you must combine your modified eating habits with exercise for two reasons. Firstly, a slender, untoned body is not your end goal and, secondly, exercise helps to eliminate those extra pounds you're losing through dieting.

Nature intended us to use our muscles. Besides, your body is designed to store energy. It doesn't just store energy for the sake of it; it stores energy so that your muscle mass will always have a reserve for optimum performance. Food, energy storage and energy expenditure are intertwined.

In today's society, many people do not need to exert themselves physically. The most demanding thing they do is get up from their desk to walk to the office coffee machine or photocopier. They have no time for sports. But they could at least walk... Some don't even have an opportunity to walk, because they drive straight from home to their place of work. Don't blame them, though; they probably have no choice.

The Subway's Pluses

Mass transit does have its advantages, as outlined in this testimonial:

"My company moved from Paris to the suburbs some time ago. Now I drive to work. Gone are my ten-minute walk to the subway station, two connections, endless corridors and countless steps... I was delighted! I wasn't as tired, arrived at work sooner and parking was free. I soon felt the consequences, though, because I gained six pounds in one year. At first I had forgotten about my daily half-hour walk and the dozens of steps that I used to go up and down. In the end, I wondered if I wouldn't be better off taking the subway because it made me exercise without my realizing it. And I don't like to exercise."

Using your muscles is natural and avoiding exercise so that you won't get tired is not always a good thing.

How do Muscles Work?

Muscles need fuel – glycogen – to work. Glycogen is stored in the liver and muscles. The body has a glycogen reserve of about 1200 calories. Once those calories are used up, the body must convert fat into glucose for fuel.

Most sports cause you to burn 500 to 600 calories per hour. So, theoretically, you'll deplete your glycogen reserves after about two hours of physical activity. As a matter of fact, fats take over in thirty minutes to provide the body with the energy it needs. Of course, how soon your body dips into that fat will depend on the type of physical activity, its intensity and its duration.

Imagine that you have 40 excess pounds; that's how much baggage you're allowed to take on an airplane. Does that mean you are always carrying those excess 40 pounds around? No, because that mass also includes the weight of your muscles. When you lose weight, you must not lose muscle. You can only "make" muscles in two ways: when you're growing and when you're exercising.

If you're well intentioned and want to get back into sports, do so with moderation unless you're already in shape. Your heart – a muscle – might be unable to handle physical exertion that exceeds its capacity. If you've been inactive for a long time, don't push yourself. Follow your nutritionist's advice based on the results of your cardiovascular function tests.

Intense physical activity may be counterproductive. The more intense the physical activity, the more glycogen your body will burn. The goal is to reduce the amount of body fat, which requires mild, regular physical activity over a long period of time. Mild physical activity is also better for your heart and figure.

Muscles are made of slow- and fast-twitch muscle fibres, whose proportions vary from one individual to another (another hereditary injustice). Fast-twitch muscle fibres are used during brief spurts of intense physical activity like sprinting, tennis or squash. Slow-twitch muscle fibres are used during lengthy and less-demanding physical activities like swimming, cycling, walking or long-distance running. You have no doubt inferred that fast-twitch muscle fibres burn up glycogen (brief, intense physical activity that does not draw on fat), while slow-twitch muscle fibres draw on fat reserves.

So, there's no point in pushing yourself to do intense physical activity to which your body is not accustomed. Mild, regular, long-term exercise will draw on your reserves while also building up your muscles, provided you do not lack proteins. If I hire a bricklayer to build a wall but don't give him any bricks (proteins), he'll be wasting his time (activity) and won't be able to build my wall. The same thing happens with physical activity. If you exercise but have no protein intake, you'll become tired and won't build up any muscle. You're basically wasting your time…

The Lasting Benefits of Physical Activity

Physical activity won't make you slim down, but it will keep you from putting on weight. It makes weight stabilization easier because it increases your energy expenditure at rest.

When you're active, you increase your energy expenditure; however, you'll need to swim or jog for hours to burn just two pounds of fat. So why do any physical activity at all if it'll improve your figure negligibly?

Toned muscles not only improve your physique, but they also continue burning calories after you've stopped exercising. Fit muscles are bulkier, and bulkier muscles require more energy. In addition, lean body mass (muscles and internal organs) acts like a "machine" that takes time to cool down. Your body will only slightly reduce the amount of calories it burns long after you've stopped exercising. A muscular body burns more energy for a longer period of time while at rest than a non-muscular body.

Be Consistent

Slowly but surely, your body will become accustomed to regularly burning more fat through its muscles because you are physically active almost every day. After a meal, calories will first be sent to the muscles to be burned up and won't be stored. A woman with a normal BMI who gets little to no exercise has about 25% body fat, while a man has about 15% body fat. Those figures drop to 10% for an active woman and to 5% for an active man.

Physical activity, whether it's a sport or some other type of activity, need not be exhausting; it just needs to be regular. Walking at a pace of about two miles an hour or at a slightly faster pace of three miles an hour will yield the same results for your body. What counts is that you walk for two hours, not that you walk briskly.

Choosing an Activity

If you already love physical activity, you certainly don't need any advice or ideas on how to find an activity that suits you. If you go to a fitness centre, a specialist can develop an exercise program for you, monitor your activity and regularly take stock of your progress with you. Fitness centres have numerous benefits: they often offer a variety of activities, have weight training equipment and give group courses that work the abs, buttocks or cardiovascular system. Some also have a swimming pool. Fitness centres also have some drawbacks: a slightly heightened atmosphere of competition (some people are disheartened by toned muscles) and their cost. Joining a fitness club is an investment that you'll want to amortize by going often.

Expand Your Horizons

There is a host of affordable, easy activities that you can do on your own wherever you want. Don't push yourself or seek performance. Focus on exercising regularly and, more importantly, have fun! Walking, swimming and cycling are fun. If you find a physical activity a chore, switch.

If you start gradually, you'll soon want to go a little farther and build up your endurance. You're basically competing with yourself at your pace.

Never underestimate the value of walking. You don't need to walk briskly or far. A good, daily walk is all you need. You don't need fancy, expensive equipment; you don't need to go to a fitness centre and follow schedules; and there's no excuse for not going for a walk.

If you feel that walking alone is not enough, pick up the pace and jog. Jogging improves your breathing and strengthens your leg, arm and back muscles. Many find that jogging is a great way to unwind. However, you'll need a good pair of jogging shoes to prevent joint pain.

Cycling, too, is an excellent physical activity that burns more than 500 calories per hour, transforms your legs into gams and strengthens your heart.

Swimming is a great gentle, basic physical activity, and prolonged contact with water is soothing. You can swim laps at a leisurely pace or give aqua fitness a try – it's fun. Aquatic workouts are low impact and can greatly reduce the injury and strain common to most land-based exercise because water acts as a cushion.

If you're under a great deal of stress, go for a gentle activity like stretching, yoga or tai chi. Don't let the gentle, harmonious movements fool you; these activities are as effective as more vigorous physical activities.

If it's fun you're looking for, there's no shortage of activities. You can skip if your apartment building has a suitable room (tenants on the floor below might not like listening to you skip and if you skip outside you may end up being the centre of unwanted attention). You may have skipped a lot as a child and now think that it's exhausting. That's why it's important to start slowly. Let your breathing guide you: stop as soon as you're out of breath. Start again the next day and gradually increase the number of skips.

Dancing is another option. Ballroom dances are an excellent physical activity that improves breathing, endurance, flexibility and posture (you always have a very upright posture when dancing). And dancing is fun. Plus, there are oodles of dances you can learn at dance studios that are more fun than ab work-outs: African dances, flamenco, jazz, tap dancing. The choices are almost endless.

Yes, but what if I stop?

What if I stop exercising? Will I become flabbier than before?

That's a risk that muscle-builders take when they pump iron to excess. If you exercise moderately on a regular basis, you won't need to worry about becoming flabby.

What if I'm hungry after a workout?

You're probably more thirsty than hungry. It's normal to drink lots of fluids after exercising, because your body has lost a great deal of water. The secret is to avoid overly sweet beverages and to go for those that are just sweet enough to provide energy. Salty drinks are better, because they replenish the salts your body has lost through perspiration.

As for appetite, you'd better rethink your preconceived notions.

Experiments on rats revealed that an active rat that became inactive sought solace by gobbling down food and getting fat, perhaps out of inactivity or to compensate for it. It turns out that the same is true for people. A sedentary lifestyle increases food intake more than regular physical activity does. When you're active, you eat fewer calories and the calories you do eat are burned faster and better.

There's an added benefit: regular exercise tends to delay weight gain, as shown by an experiment conducted in 1995. Two groups of obese women were put on a diet, but only one group exercised. The women who exercised had an easier time sticking to their diet and once their diet ended, 90% of them maintained their new weight, compared to just 34% of the women in the group that did not exercise. An excellent example, don't you think?

16 Recap

The quick, long-lasting, weight-
loss method can be summed up in
a few lines.

Phase 1: The Protein Diet

Goal: force your body to live off its reserves by burning fat, while conserving proteins and giving the pancreas a rest.

Diet: protein packets in different flavours that are mixed with water, and unlimited vegetables.

Possibly: white meat or fish once a day, accompanied with vegetables, depending on your nutritionist's instructions.

Duration: duration varies from one individual to another. It depends on the amount of pounds to be lost and your nutritionist's opinion.

Result: women lose 8 to 10 pounds in three weeks, while men lose 10 to 12 pounds (these figures are for reference purposes only and may vary significantly).

Transition Phases

The protein diet does not end with the stabilization phase. Calories, fats and carbohydrates are gradually reintroduced to your diet during successive phases. Remember that deep-sea diver who makes decompression stops during his ascent? You're in a similar situation if you go on the protein diet, because you can't go back to eating normally at all once.

The intermediate phases are established with your nutritionist. It's hard to generalize, given the differences among patients.

Phase 2: The Stabilization Phase

Goal: maintain your ideal weight, while continuing to go easy on the pancreas which secretes insulin in order to control the sugar level in the bloodstream.

Principles:

            - balance is achieved over a 24-hour period and not

on a meal-by-meal basis.

- fats and carbohydrates are not eaten during the same meal. Proteins do not need to be separated from other food groups.

Diet:

• Breakfast (carbohydrates + proteins):

- a slice of lightly buttered, whole-wheat bread, possibly with lightly sweetened or fructose-sweetened jam, or cereal;

- a dairy product: yogurt, cottage cheese, hard cheese from time to time;

- a beverage: coffee or tea or an infusion;

- perhaps a fruit.

• Lunch (mostly proteins):

- lean meat or fish, or eggs;

- unlimited vegetables;

- yogurt or cheese (optional).

• Snack (optional):

- a fruit, yogurt, or a whole-wheat muffin with two pieces of chocolate.

• Dinner:

- 150 to 200 g of complex carbohydrates, weighed and cooked;

- unlimited vegetables;

- a not-too-sweet dessert or a fruit;

- perhaps lean proteins (an egg, a slice of ham, a small filet of fish) only if you absolutely can't do without them.

<u>Duration:</u> as long as possible. In fact, you can eat this way as long as you like. Frustrated? Not if you've learned how to manage those diet slips.

Careful!

Although the protein diet results in fast, efficient weight loss, its true effects will be felt after a long, in-depth period of nutritional rehabilitation. It is important that you do not skip the stabilization phase and that you stay on it as long as possible.

Why would you risk skipping this phase? Because the initial weight loss is so fast that patients are not always fully aware of how they must fundamentally change their eating habits. Only on this point are the method's detractors right… just a little.

Remember the main points:

- eat complex carbohydrates every evening;

- do not combine carbohydrates and fats in a single meal;

- learn to manage your diet slip-ups;

- ignore those who are jealous or who make ironical comments;

- exercise.

These simple, easy-to-remember tips will help you to control your weight as efficiently and easily as possible.

17 Frequently Asked Questions

Is the diet harmful in any way?

The protein-sparing diet is not an aggressive weight-loss method, because it involves no medication. It's not a high protein diet, because you eat the proteins your body actually needs and no more. Therefore, it does not affect the kidneys more than any other protein diet consisting of meat, fish, eggs and dairy products.

- Do not go on a high-protein diet if you have severe impairment in kidney function.

- Do not go on the protein diet if you have insulin-dependent diabetes mellitus, not because of the proteins but because of the sugars that are eliminated.

- If you've recently had a cardiovascular incident, do not go on an overly strict diet of any kind.

- The protein diet is not for children who haven't finished growing, nor is it for pregnant or breastfeeding women. Any effective diet results in a deficiency that proteins cannot correct.

- The main hazard of protein diets is a potassium deficiency, which can be harmful to your heart. That's why you need blood work and monitoring by a nutritionist.

Hundreds of thousands of people follow the protein diet every year. No incident has been recorded in the more than twelve years the diet has been used in France. The same cannot be said for other weight-loss treatments. Should there ever be an incident, it'll most likely be due to failure by therapists-turned-nutritionists to follow the protocol's basic rules or to self-medication.

How long does the protein diet take?

The protein diet is not a long-term diet. It generally takes twenty days and may be prolonged in some cases. Your diet will be tailored to you, because you don't have the same pounds to lose as someone else and because you put them on under different circumstances. Your age, family circumstance and health status affect the treatment and its length.

When will I start to see results?

Results vary, depending on your gender, metabolism and starting weight. During the first week, you'll lose two to six pounds of water due to diuresis. So, if you lose six pounds during the first week, don't be alarmed. Weight loss will be less spectacular in the weeks that follow. After three weeks, you'll be well on your way to losing weight: a woman loses about eight pounds during that timeframe. At that point, you must assess your situation and decide to continue with the protein diet under the supervision of a nutritionist or move on to the pre-stabilization phase during which you will continue to lose weight. Your nutritionist will gradually decrease the number of protein packets and reintroduce natural proteins. Since the protein diet corrects the way your body (especially the pancreas) reacts to food, your cravings for a sugar fix will be reduced.

What will I be eating?

Your diet consists of:

- protein packets (3 to 4 per day);

- unlimited raw or cooked vegetables, with or without herbs, spices and seasoning, one tablespoon of olive, canola or sunflower oil per day, to make up for the essential fatty acid deficiency;

- lean meat or fish once a day:

- Lean fish: any white fish, such as sole, dab (a flatfish), turbot, pollack…. So-called "blue" fish are not allowed because of their high fat content: mackerel, tuna, salmon…;

- Lean meat: white chicken or turkey meat, veal scallop, lean ham, guinea fowl.

You must simply do without other foods, because they contain varying amounts of carbohydrates and fat.

You won't be eating any of these foods during Phase 1:

- deli meats, eggs, dairy products (cheese, cottage cheese, yogurt, butter, cream);

- all cereals and starchy foods: bread and all bread products (rusk, melba toast), potatoes, rice, pasta, pulses;

- all fats: oil (except a tablespoon per day), butter, fresh cream (do not add any cream to the protein packets or oil to your crudités);

- all fruits;

- anything sweet: pastries, candies, cookies, store-bought desserts – including sugar-free, fat-free desserts – (you can make your own desserts using protein packets), chocolate, jam.

It is important to stay away from all foods that'll make you gain weight AND that'll stall the weight loss. All foods listed above may not make you gain weight, but they will keep you from losing it.

I'm afraid the protein diet will be difficult...

You may be tormented by irrepressible cravings for a "forbidden fruit" during the first two to three days of the diet when *ketosis* is induced. Hang in there and don't succumb to a food that'll keep you from losing weight (that would be like starting over, because you'll stop *ketosis*). You'll soon be rewarded: the diet will seem easier, because you will have become accustomed to doing without certain foods (you were probably addicted to sugar) and because *ketosis* releases substances similar to amphetamines, which are natural appetite suppressants and boost your energy level and enthusiasm. This is a major plus. Every time you step on the weigh scale you'll see that the diet is worth the effort.

Although the diet may be difficult, it is of limited duration. It'll be over before you know it, especially given the very long-term benefits.

I don't find the protein packets appealing. Can't I eat foods that contain protein?

You could lose weight without the protein packets, but you would not get the same results. You could even lose weight without using a single packet (isn't that how people lost weight before?). However, to lose weight safely without harming your muscles and vital organs, you need to provide your body with all of the essential amino acids it needs. And when we say all essential amino acids, we mean all essential amino acids, and not those found in a cod filet or yogurt. When you're on a diet, your muscles and organs (like your heart) are more at risk than when you are not on a diet, because they are made of protein. Food provides carbohydrates, which are your body's main fuel and prevent muscles from melting away.

You could theoretically combine various protein-containing foods when you're on a diet. For your diet to be complete, you'd have to combine animal and plant proteins. However, animal proteins are always associated with varying amounts of fat, while plant proteins are always associated with carbohydrates. There is no pure, isolated protein that is complete. That's why it's safer and easier to use an ideally reconstituted protein which contains all amino acids. It's the best way to obtain the most protein with the fewest calories.

It's easier to use protein packets than to spend your time trying to figure out which foods you should combine to obtain the right combination of essential amino acids while keeping the calories down.

Are all proteins created equally?

Let's make a distinction between high-protein preparations and so-called balanced meal replacements, which are supposed to contain fewer calories than a normal meal. Meal replacements, which are even sold in superstores, contain a large amount of sugar, which prevents efficient weight loss (*ketosis*). Their only focus is to be low-calorie.

High-protein preparations are strictly regulated and contain virtually no sugar. They must have a perfect composition of essential amino acids in very precise proportions, known as their chemical score. Two powders containing the same proportion of proteins do not necessarily have the same biological value, because their essential amino acid content and efficacy may be different.

The first proteins used in the United States in the 1970s had a very low biological value. Nowadays, quality control is very strict and most proteins have satisfactory specifications.

I strongly discourage protein preparations that contain animal gelatin or gelatin obtained from GM foods, such as genetically modified soybeans.

Can any high-protein preparation be used during a protein diet, as long as its protein content is high and sugar content is low?

Fitness buffs who are heavily into body-building have been using high-protein preparations for years. These products are not strictly controlled systematically and most are not regulatory.

Remember that body-builders who eat these proteins already have a very rich diet. So, if the protein has a minor deficiency, it will have no consequences.

A person on the protein diet exclusively eats certain proteins instead of a regular diet; therefore, a deficiency in the proteins may have significant health consequences. So, follow the advice of your nutritionist who will give you proteins with full knowledge of your situation.

Do the packets contain artificial protein?

Not any more than infant formula. The protein you are given is not artificial and is reconstituted from natural ingredients.

What about my social life? Should I give up dining with friends?

While you're on the protein diet, say good-bye to invitations that you give out or receive, do not eat at your workplace restaurant or at any other restaurant for that matter. Stick to your protein packets, vegetables, crudités, and lean meat or fish once a day.

Put your social life on hold, keeping the following in mind: you're not just going on a diet that allows slips; you're undergoing a therapeutic process. This concept is important: you are being treated for a (pancreatic) dysfunction that resulted in overweight. When you are ill and seek treatment, you don't feel like having an exciting social life. You follow your treatment and get better. Once you've recovered, you can resume your social activities.

Of course, you're not sick because none of your other activities has changed and you even feel great, but keep in mind that while you're on the protein diet, you're under treatment.

Why this diet instead of another?

Because this diet lets you kill two birds with one stone. First, you retain your muscle mass, which is your body's motor. Consequently, you "burn" as much energy after the diet as before, which is not the case with low-calorie diets that inevitably increasingly reduce muscle mass – a major calorie burner – as time goes on.

Second, your pancreas rests while you're on the diet. It'll be regenerated and repair itself. It'll function better for better weight stabilization.

What are the diet's conditions?

The first condition is that you must use protein packets during the Phase 1. These substitutes are reconstituted food and not natural food. Don't kid yourself: although most of the protein packets are delicious and can be enhanced in different ways, they do not lend themselves to great culinary feats.

And you have to buy them, which means you must order them or purchase them at a point of sale. Be sure stock a good supply so that you won't run out.

Is it more expensive? Not necessarily. The protein packets should not cost more than regular foods. Remember that you won't need to buy bread, cheese, meat, pastries, wine, alcohol, crackers, prepared dishes, etc. You save on foods that make you gain weight (munchies) and on basic foods (meat, fish) because you eat less of them.

Some popular anti-obesity drugs are supposed to fight fat absorption. These treatments, which complement a diet, don't come cheap...

Are there other drawbacks or side effects?

Bad breath is a minor, unpleasant consequence of protein diets. To partially neutralize bad breath, eat your protein preparation first and then your vegetables. Three radishes and a celery stick or a breath spray will do the trick. Stay away from sugar-free candies which contain only carbohydrates. Read the insert carefully.

To control hypotension (which may occur during any weight-loss diet) increase your salt and water intake.

You may experience constipation due to a lack of fibre. This can easily be corrected by drinking plenty of fluids, increasing your fibre intake and perhaps using a mild laxative. Remember, there's not much in your digestive tract while you're on the protein diet.

Headaches, night cramps and intolerance to cold are other side effects that dissipate in a few days, as does the impression of weakness which can be corrected by taking potassium.

You menstrual cycle may change, as it would if you were on any other diet. Your body is adjusting to weight loss and will adapt to its new weight.

What should I do after I've completed the protein diet?

After you've completed the protein diet and lost your first pounds and after *ketosis* has begun, you may gradually reintroduce carbohydrates and fat to your diet, and then move on to the stabilization phase (see Chapter 10).

Do I run the risk of backsliding or experiencing the rebound effect?

The protein diet is often criticized for its rebound effect. But what is the rebound effect? It's an illogical effect that occurs when a treatment is suddenly stopped (tricyclic antidepressants, sleeping pills or cortisone, for example). That does not happen with the protein diet. When you go off a diet and you're not in the stabilization phase and you eat what you want when you want, you'll obviously put the pounds back on. But that's not the rebound effect; it's a normal result, a natural process, because your body is designed to store energy rather than to draw on it. You know that you "burn" fewer calories after you've been on a low-calorie diet; therefore, you might regain weight more quickly. That's a rebound effect associated with treatment cessation. The rebound effect is an inappropriate term when used in connection with the protein diet, provided you remain vigilant and don't overeat under the pretext that you've slimmed down. No diet is final and no diet can guarantee that you'll keep the weight off in the long term. The result depends on you and only you.

CONCLUSION

A hypothesis was advanced at the beginning of this book: the protein diet is one of the solutions to overweight. At the end of the day, it is THE solution. The protein diet has a thirty-year proven track record and its concept has been refined over the years. The body's needs are now better met and it is forced to use up its fat reserves.

Up until now, if you wanted to lose weight, you had only two options: eat less or eat better.

Eating less harms your muscles and almost systematically results in the lost pounds being regained.

Eating a better or more balanced diet is great if you want to maintain an appropriate weight, but it won't help you shed unwanted pounds. By definition, balance is a state of equilibrium. If you want to lose weight, you must create a monitored imbalance for a limited period of time. If you want to lose weight, you must take an unbalanced diet approach that does not harm your body and especially not your muscles. Finally, the weight loss must be long-lasting.

And then there's the other way – the method you just learned about. Although the principle is simple – taking the unbalanced diet approach to a slimmer you – it certainly gave rise to suspicion and overreaction in the conventional diet community that is incapable of changing its ways or re-examining itself. And what have we observed?

In Europe in general and in France in particular, most patients who decide to lose weight choose the protein diet. The protein diet is used the most in France, where patients are the most numerous and hungry for answers.

The time has come to demonstrate that the protein diet is the only truly effective way to attain and maintain an appropriate weight. Everyone who has lost weight by using this method unfailingly sings its praises and applauds its innocuousness and efficacy, even when it comes to stabilizing their new weight.

Is this just a craze? A fad? Perhaps. What fad can brag that it has lasted thirty years? Jeans, maybe…

APPENDICES

Appendix 1:
The Big Three: Proteins, Carbohydrates and Fats 133

Appendix 2:
Understanding the Glycemic Index 145

Appendix 3:
GI: Your Last Diet! 149

The Big Three:
Proteins, Carbohydrates and Fats

To chefs and cooks, the ingredients of delicious, flavourful dishes are foods, while nutritionists talk of nutrients and place all foods in three categories: proteins, carbohydrates or sugars, and fats.

All foods contain a combination of the big three and other components, of which the first and foremost is a varying amount of water. Dry foods (rice, pasta, flour, lentils, dried mushrooms) are simply uneatable if they haven't been hydrated or rehydrated.

Other foods, especially vegetables, contain varying amounts of fibre.

Finally, foods also contain small amounts of vitamins and trace minerals that are essential for our health.

What do we need to live? Well, all of the above, but for different purposes. Proteins, carbohydrates, fats, water, fibre, vitamins and trace minerals help our body to function properly and keep us alive.

Your body cannot do without any of these nutrients for long. Everyone knows that their diet must contain all nutrients to avoid deficiencies that will weaken their immune system, make them more susceptible to disease and diminish their vitality. Animals cannot live without food and we are animals. Plants, on the other hand, synthesize their food from minerals in the soil, carbon dioxide in the air, and sunlight.

The concept of a balanced diet must temporally be discarded during a strict diet and especially during the protein diet, because you must take the unbalanced diet approach to a slimmer you. Protein, vitamin and mineral salt supplements are essential during the short-term protein diet in order to prevent deficiencies.

Nutritionists always find it odd that many patients still find these concepts vague and somewhat confusing. There's no time like the present to top up your knowledge.

THE ROLE OF PROTEINS

Although proteins are a body's building blocks, their role is not only a structural one. Proteins are found in the cells that make up our organs and in cell membranes. Muscles, the liver, kidneys, the brain, viscera, skin, nails and hair, etc. are all made up of different proteins.

Other proteins function as enzymes, hormones and antibodies. These functional proteins help carry out activities and functions in the human body during normal and crisis situations by passing on instructions from the brain.

Amino acids – the building blocks from which proteins are constructed – number twenty. The human body can synthesize some amino acids by breaking down other amino acids, but is unable to synthesize eight essential amino acids which must be supplied by the diet. Amino acids form chains of varying complexity that make up a protein.

These twenty amino acids are common to all living things (plants, animals, humans), but their order varies for each species, determining its signature as it were.

We always need proteins. Why is our initial supply of protein insufficient after we've finished growing? Well, because things wear out…

Organs must continually replace worn tissue in order to function properly, as the body destroys about three hundred grams of its own protein every day. Even if it reconstitutes some of those proteins by breaking down other amino acids, it still needs a constant supply of proteins. Since humans cannot synthesize the essential elements it needs like plants do with nitrogen and carbon dioxide, it has to get proteins from food.

Our organs are primarily made up of proteins, but the body has no protein reserves on which it can draw (but it does have fat reserves). Proteins must be eaten regularly, almost on a daily basis; otherwise, worn tissue might not be renewed. That's why diets that are totally deficient in proteins must be regarded with suspicion. Although such diets are no longer recommended, absolute fasts and fruit diets have destroyed a great many muscles.

Which foods contain the most proteins? You already know the answer to that question: animal products, meat, dairy products, deli meats, fish and eggs all contain about 15 to 30 grams of protein per 100 grams. These complete animal proteins can easily be assimilated and are always associated with fats.

Some plants, grains and legumes also contain a fair amount of proteins. Plant proteins are always associated with carbohydrates. When combined, grains and legumes provide a high-quality protein combination.

Our body needs the proteins contained in food to function. But be careful – you don't build muscles by eating protein. Proteins only repair worn tissue.

There are only two ways to develop muscles: during growth up until adulthood and by exercising to keep your body in shape. Clearly, a minimum of muscular effort, walking, physical effort or sports is essential.

THE ROLE OF CARBOHYDRATES

Proteins are the body's building blocks, while carbohydrates are the fuel that keeps it running. Carbohydrates are also found in tissues and are essential for nerve cells.

Where do carbohydrates come from? They mostly come from plants. Like their name implies, carbohydrates contain water and carbon and are produced by photosynthetic plants.

Every time you eat carbohydrates, they're used immediately (glucose) or stored as glycogen in the liver and muscles for future use. Your body has a fifteen-hour supply of energy. And if you have far too much energy, it becomes fat.

Glucose – a ready source of energy – circulates in the blood and needs insulin in order to penetrate cells that need energy. Glycogen, however, is a more basic reserve, but can be released very quickly when necessary.

There are many types of carbohydrates, some of which cannot be assimilated and are thus termed unavailable: fibre that passes through the small intestine without being converted and is eliminated as waste, providing the body with virtually no calories.

There are numerous available carbohydrates (sugars).

- Monosaccharides, or simple sugars, have that pleasant, sweet taste. Monosaccharides include glucose (the perfect sweet sugar) and fructose (present in fruit). These sugars do not need to be digested and go directly into the bloodstream, which is why they are erroneously called fast sugars, a well-known term that is rapidly becoming obsolete.

- Disaccharides, or sugars composed of two monosaccharides, include sucrose (from sugar cane or sugar beets, for example) which is sold in supermarkets, and lactose (present in milk and milk products).

- Polysaccharides, or complex sugars, are chains consisting of a number of monosaccharides. Polysaccharides include starch (which gives cereals their texture), pulses and starchy foods. Complex sugars are digested more slowly, are not sweet-tasting and are called slow sugars because of the amount of time they spend in the digestive tract.

When you eat sugar, glycemia – or the presence of glucose in the blood – increases measurably and that increase is measured by the glycemic index.

A food that contains a slow sugar that takes time to enter the bloodstream will affect glycemia only slightly, causing a lower and more gentle change in blood sugar. Consequently, it has a low glycemic index.

Conversely, a food that is rich in fast sugars will cause your blood sugar to spike rapidly. It is classified as having a high glycemic index.

Insulin helps to transport glucose from your food into cells where it is burned, thereby lowering the blood glucose level.

The concept of fast and slow sugars is fairly easy to remember. But things are not really that simple. Some sugars should logically be slow. Take the sugars in white bread: they act like fast sugars that quickly enter the bloodstream. Even table sugar is slightly slower than the sugars in white bread. What is a person to do?

Furthermore, the more a food is ground up, the higher its glycemic index (because it can be digested more quickly and easily). Lentil puree has a higher glycemic index than plain lentils. So, don't grind or break up your foods to avoid increasing their glycemic index. Your figure will thank you.

If you know a food's glycemic index, you'll be able to determine if it's allowed on the protein diet or during the maintenance phase, and you'll be able to watch what you eat each day. (See the Glycemic Index in Appendix 2 which lists the foods you're most likely to encounter in your daily life.)

Must you forego fast, blissfully sweet sugars forever? These sugars and white bread taste great, but don't forget that they're often combined with fat (chocolate, pastries). It's a disastrous combination for very emotional people. Fast carbohydrates do boost energy quickly when necessary, while the body waits for slow sugars to kick in. However, it's always better to choose slow sugars, snack on a whole-wheat muffin instead of cake, and skip the chocolate.

Sugar, My Daily Drug

Unlike other classes of food, sugar holds a special meaning for people. Sugar is ambiguous, because it's both a danger and a pleasure. There's no escaping it; sugar is a drug, especially (but not only) fast sugar on its own or in a mixture (pastry, chocolate), which has a characteristic, distinct taste. Carbohydrates are just not sweet enough. Once they become accustomed to sugar, our taste buds can't do without its pleasant taste.

Habituation – a desire to increase doses, strong attraction – and the fact that pure sugar is not found in nature, make sugar a drug. The taste for sugar – which unfortunately makes us gain weight without a way out – is spontaneous. You can't help but like sugar the very first time it lands on your tongue. Other drugs are different: the first alcoholic beverage or the first cigarette is not that great. Once you've forced yourself to like alcohol or tobacco, you can become "addicted". Sugar is different.

An Early, Wide-spread Pleasure

Take a newborn who has not yet had its first nursing and has no sense of taste and give him four nipples dipped in products corresponding to the four basic tastes: sweet, salty, sour, bitter.

When his lips and tongue touch the salty, bitter and sour nipples, he pulls away his tongue, turns his head and shows his disgust. He's clearly not happy. Give him a sugary nipple and he'll vigorously and blissfully suck on it. He definitely likes it and soon he'll ask for more.

What can be done to counter such an early, spontaneous and natural taste for sugar that is so bad? You try to understand it, curb it and go without in, but in vain.

Humans are not the only victims of sugar. Most animals, from horses to ants, wasps to dogs and hummingbirds to tigers, like all things sweet.

Sugar as a Reward or Consolation and Its Emotional Ties

The field of psychology quickly weighed in. Every individual's upbringing is somehow connected with sugar. It's almost unavoidable.

As children develop, they learn a simple equation that they won't soon forger: sugar equals pleasure and reward. Repeated negative and positive reinforcement ("no dessert for you" or "you can have one candy") firmly fixes the process in the sub-consciousness, so that it can be called upon as soon as is there the slightest emotional or ego weakness.

Not too long ago, sugar was not particularly scarce or exotic, but it was not a ubiquitous product either.

A morning coffee with two sugars, yogurt with a spoonful of sugar instead of a fruit for dessert, Sunday cake, candies as a reward, a piece of comforting chocolate to smooth life's bumps, lollipops brought by visitors, candies for Christmas.

While they were considered rewards, sweets had a reputation of spoiling children (not to mention that it ruined their teeth). Then the moralizers stepped in and primarily linked gluttony – a deadly sin – with a strong, natural craving for sweets.

Sugar, Sugar Everywhere

Times have changed. Affordable sugar is now found in count-less common food products to which children – and many adults – are partial. Oodles of milk products, like yogurt, mousse, ice cream, cream, custard pies, clafoutis, rice pudding and floating islands, have become French children's favourite twice-daily dessert, at the expense of less-sweet fruit which contain more vitamins and nutrients, but that are hard to keep, often a hassle to peel and balked at by children.

A milk dessert is the best and easiest dessert.

There's a dizzying array of store-bought cakes, cookies and pastries. Some may claim to contain vitamins and other ingredients that are healthy or good for growing children, but the fact remains that their main ingredients are slow and fast sugars and fat. That does not bode well for the figures of future adults or for their nutritional education, because they may find it unbearable to limit these desserts.

Add to that the ever-widening range of drinks, fruit juices, sodas and syrups, and the sugar needlessly added to all kinds of prepared foods (salads, crackers, savoury pies) and it's obvious that temptation is everywhere.

An Antidepressant

Under these conditions, it's difficult to inform people about dietetics and especially about reasonable sugar consumption.

When sweetness is enhanced by a velvety, melt-in-your mouth fat, you have the ultimate danger: pastries and chocolate.

Chocolate – an antidepressant – makes the blues and difficulties easier to handle not only because its taste reminds you of your childhood, but also because of the magnesium and theobromine it contains which help you fight fatigue and overcome difficulties. Lentils (carbohydrates, magnesium) have the same effect, but they certainly don't offer chocolate's taste.

Chocolate ends up causing a new type of depression: that associated with extra pounds caused by a combination of fast sugars and fat deposited in fat cells.

Like alcoholics, "chocoholics" bite into a chocolate bar or a praline cluster to forget that they gained weight. They console themselves by saying it's their only remaining pleasure. They have no desire to lose weight, because they'd have to give up their delicious drug.

Those who want to get back their slim figure find it excruciatingly difficult to give up chocolate. But if they're determined, they'll succeed, knowing better than anyone else that you don't get something for nothing.

THE ROLE OF FATS

Proteins and carbohydrates have four calories per gram, while fats have nine.

Remember that your body is designed to store fat rather than to burn it and that long, long ago fats were a tremendous safety net because they provide more energy per volume. It's always good to eat fat when food is scarce, isn't it?

Our affluent society loves to hate fats, but fats are essential.

Fats are essential to fine cooking, because they give foods their unctuous, soft texture, impart a smooth and lustrous look to dishes, make it possible to brown foods and give fries their crunch. Fats also exude and fix the aroma of dishes, enhance dishes and make their flavour linger in the mouth. (Perfume makers steep flowers in a very pure fat to extract and fix their highly volatile fragrant oils.)

Everything that is creamy and melts in your mouth contains fat. It's hard to go without fat if you're a food aficionado or a foodie. If you eliminate all fats from your diet, you'll have to resign yourself to eating bland, boring foods that are an organoleptic desert.

Fats are not only essential for gastronomy, but they also play a vital biological role.

Fats provide heat; they protect us from temperature fluctuations in the outside world and are an excellent thermal insulation. If you had no fat, you'd be a walking skeleton. Fats also form a protective layer around organs. They shape your body and make it soft and curvy. Although it's sometimes difficult to maintain a balanced fat intake, opting for a totally fat-free diet would be a tragic error.

Fats play a vital role in blood coagulation and tissue regeneration and are particularly important for neural tissue and the brain.

They help transport certain fat-soluble vitamins: vitamins A, D, E and K. The more fat, the more vitamins are supplied.

Fats contain essential fatty acids, some of which your body cannot make and must be supplied by the diet.

Although fats can be eliminated while you're on a diet, it's impossible to go without them totally. Besides, your social life would suffer immensely.

The Structure of Fats

The fats occurring naturally in foods are triglycerides, the molecules of which consist of a combination of glycerol and three fatty acids.

There are three kinds of fatty acids and all are vital for our body.

Saturated fatty acids occur naturally in animal fat: meat, egg yolk, and milk and dairy products, including butter. Excessive consumption of saturated fatty acids will result in elevated blood cholesterol and clog arteries. Fat carried by the blood forms plaques (atheromas) in and beneath the inner lining of arterial walls, narrowing arteries slowly but surely, and may cause serious vascular disorders. This medical condition is worsened by smoking, stress and genetics.

There are two categories of unsaturated fatty acids: monounsaturated and polyunsaturated.

Monounsaturated fatty acids are found mainly in three oils: canola, olive and peanut oil. They reduce bad cholesterol without affecting good cholesterol. The fatty acids they contain are not essential, meaning that the body can synthesize them.

Polyunsaturated fatty acids are found in such oils as grape seed, canola and sunflower oil, margarine and fish. They reduce bad cholesterol (the artery-clogging type caused by saturated fatty acids) and good cholesterol, which protects against heart attacks. These oils go rancid quickly and are dangerous if rancid.

Some polyunsaturated fatty acids cannot be synthesized by the human body and must therefore be supplied by the diet.

A balanced diet requires you to alternate between sources of fatty acids, vary pleasures and not limit yourself to one category. These principles can be applied to all foods, because you need to eat a little of everything every day.

WHAT ABOUT VEGETABLES?

Into which category do vegetables fall? They are not sweet, fat or rich in protein.

Let's put them in the fibre category. Green vegetables primarily consist of water and indigestible fibre that passes through the digestive tract in order to facilitate the transit of waste, releasing the vitamins and trace minerals it contains. Vegetable fibre is made of "unavailable" carbohydrates. Most vegetables contain a negligible amount of "available" carbohydrates.

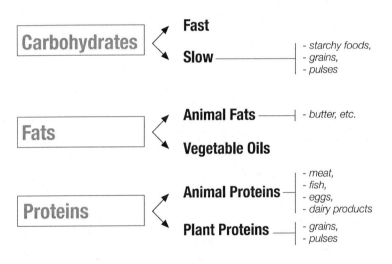

UNDERSTANDING
THE GLYCEMIC INDEX

In this book, a distinction is made between fast and slow sugars.

- Fast sugars are defined as simple carbohydrates that are easily and quickly absorbed by the body. For example:

  Glucose, which is not a food in itself;
  Sucrose (glucose + fructose) or table sugar;
  Fructose, a sugar that occurs naturally in fruit;
  Lactose, a sugar that occurs naturally in milk (glucose + galactose);
  Maltose, the sugar found in beer (glucose + glucose).

- Slow sugars such as starch are carbohydrates with a complex molecular structure, which are absorbed more slowly by the body than simple sugars.

  Starchy foods, grains and legumes all contain starch.

It turns out that not all fast sugars are "bad" and that not all slow sugars are necessarily good.

In fact, some complex sugars can cause blood sugar levels to spike faster than some simple sugars can.

For example, a baked potato will cause a faster rise in blood sugar than a fruit or honey will.

These observations have led doctors to create a new system for classifying carbohydrates called the GLYCEMIC INDEX.

Developed in the 1980s, the glycemic index classifies carbohydrate-containing foods based on their ability to raise blood sugar levels, or glycemia. Foods are ranked on a scale of 0 to 100 based on how much glucose they produce in the blood in relation to a reference food.

There are two classifications depending on the reference food.

In France, glucose is the reference food and its glycemic index (GI) is arbitrarily set at 100. Glycemic index values for different foods are calculated by comparing measurements of their effects on blood glucose at an equal carbohydrate portion of glucose.

A baked potato has a GI of 95; white bread, 85 (sandwich bread and not a baguette); honey, 90; whole brown rice, 45; quinoa, 35; grapefruit, 22, etc....

In North America, white bread is the reference food; it has a GI of 100. All other foods are compared to white bread rather than glucose, which is actually not a food in itself.

Why is it important to know a food's glycemic index?

When you eat something sweet, your blood sugar level rises. Two parameters affect by how much and how quickly the blood sugar level rises:

- The amount of sugar absorbed;

- The type of sugar.

As you know, an increase in the blood sugar level causes insulin to be secreted into the bloodstream.

Insulin is the key that opens a cell so that blood sugar can enter it. That sugar is stored as glycogen in the liver and muscles.

Once a cell's sugar needs are exceeded, insulin turns into a formidable hormone that causes excess sugar to be stored as fat in the fat cells. The result is weight gain at first and then a malfunctioning pancreas, which can lead to a collection of illnesses called metabolic syndrome or Syndrome X:

Abdominal obesity, cardiovascular events, high blood pressure, type 2 diabetes, hyperlipidemia.

What about those low-GI diets?

The glycemic index was initially intended to help diabetics plan their diet, by recommending that they select low-GI foods and avoid wide blood glucose fluctuations.

Gradually, many authors started to recommend weight-loss diets based on the GI, which have become the flavour of the month.

I have certain reservations regarding this approach.

Obviously, if you're overweight and have a very poor diet that is high in "bad sugars", you can lose weight just by improving your diet and replacing high-GI carbohydrates with low-GI carbohydrates. This method will also make you more aware of healthy practices. If it was that easy, you could stop at that. But unfortunately, that is not the case. Many overweight individuals do not necessarily eat a great deal, much less bad sugars, but they just can't take off the pounds because their metabolism is too "lazy" and their pancreas is not functioning properly. The GI method will be of no help to them; only the protein diet with an initial reduction in the amount of all good and bad sugars will yield results. The concept of GI is used later on during the maintenance phase and to teach these individuals about good eating habits.

Remember, just because you're not gaining weight doesn't mean you're losing weight!

To lose weight, you must avoid the foods that cause you to gain weight and the foods that keep you from taking the pounds off. And low-GI foods keep you from losing weight.

I continue to separate fast and slow sugars, because I think that food combinations are more important than their GI.

A look at glycemic indices raises some questions:

The glycemic index of rice flour pasta is (95) and higher than that of honey (90), sweet white wines (90), gummy candies (80), pound cake (75), champagne (70), table sugar, (sucrose, 65), cookies (60), and ice cream (60)!

Rice flour pasta is an essential part of the daily diet in the Far East, and until there is proof to the contrary, obesity has not reached endemic proportions in that region!

GI: YOUR LAST DIET!

HIGH GI FOODS
BAD SUGARS

110	Beer, maltose and malto-dextrins Doughnuts
100	Glucose
95	Potatoes, baked or steamed French fries Puffed rice cakes Rice flour pasta Flans Cooked wines, including port wine
90	Potatoes, mashed White rice, quick cooking Honey White wine, sweet Kir
85	Overly cooked pasta Carrots, cooked Cornflakes and corn cereals Popcorn White bread Cider Rice pudding
80	Beans and chestnuts Gummy candies Gingerbread Crackers Swedish rolls No sugar added pineapple juice Tapioca

75 Winter squash
Baguette
Waffles
Pound cake
Weetabix®
Coco Pops®
Rosé wine
Watermelon

70 Croissants
Scones
Gnocchi
Country bread
Sugary cereals, not corn-based
Chocolate bars
Potatoes, boiled in their skin
Corn
Corn starch
Turnips
Soft drinks
No sugar added grapefruit juice
Champagne

65 Potatoes, peeled and boiled
Beets
White semolina (couscous and tabbouleh)
Sucrose: sweets and candies
Cereal bars
Bananas, pineapple, melon
Raisins, dates, prunes, dried figs, nuts
(hazelnuts, pistachios, almonds...)
Jams
Orange juice, commercial

60 Papaya
Chips
Cookies
No sugar added apple juice
Ice cream

MEDIUM GI FOODS
BETTER SUGARS

55   Biscuits ("Social Tea" or shortbread)
       Muesli
       Diet cereals
       Kiwis
       Orange juice, fresh
       Peaches, in syrup
       Jams, light
       Grain bread

50   Whole wheat bread
       Rolled oats
       Buckwheat
       Dark chocolate, less than 70% cocoa
       Muffins, apple
       Basmati rice, Thai rice and wild rice
       Green peas, canned
       Carrots, raw
       Sweet potatoes
       Dry pasta, cooked al dente
       Mango and other exotic fruit
       Sherbet
       Red wine and dry white wine

LOW GI FOODS
BEST SUGARS

45   Whole brown rice
       Whole wheat semolina
       Ebly® Tender Wheat
       Bulgur wheat
       Pasta, fresh
       Red kidney beans
       Bran and rye bread
       Porridge
       Green peas, fresh
       Grapes
       Oranges

	Peaches, canned
	Pears, canned
40	Plums
35	Whole wheat pasta
	Quinoa
	Chinese vermicelli
	Stone-ground whole wheat bread
	Fish sticks
	Jams, sweetened with fructose
	Yogurt
	Apples and pears
	Apricots, dried
	Figs, fresh
30	Beans, dried (flageolets, white kidney beans)
	Chick peas
	Lentils, brown
	Green beans
	Wax beans
	Peaches
	No sugar added fruit marmalade
	Milk
	Chocolate milk, unsweetened
22	Split peas
	Green lentils
	Cherries
	Grapefruit
	Chocolate, more than 70% cocoa
20	Fructose
	Peanuts
	Soya
	Apricots
	Nuts
	All vegetables (including tomatoes)
	Onions
	Garlic and green onions
	Red fruit (strawberries, gooseberries, raspberries....)
	Spirits, dry, not sweetened to taste

BIBLIOGRAPHY

General Book:

HARRISON, T.R. *Principes de médecine interne.* Flammarion, Petit Larousse de la médecine, Larousse, 2002.

Nutrition and Diet Books:

ADRIAN J., J.J. BERNIER, B. GUY-GRAND, A. MOUTON, G. PASCAL, P. PYNSON, D. RIGAUD. *Nutrition à la carte, de l'aliment au métabolisme.* Institut Danone, 1993.

APFELDORFER, G. *Maigrir, c'est fou !* Odile Jacob, 2000.

ATKINS, R.C. *La révolution diététique du D' Atkins.* Buchat-Chastel, 1975.

ATKINSO, C. *Cuisine pour rester mince.* La Cuisine Illustrée, 1999.

BLACKBURN, G.L., G.A. BRAY, *Management of obesity by severe caloric restriction.* PSG Publishing CO., Littleton, Mass., USA, 1985.

CORCOS, M. *Le corps absent. Approche psychosomatique des troubles des conduites alimentaires.* Dunod, 2000.

DUFOUR, A. *Régimes, toute la vérité. 101 idées fausses et 101 réponses justes.* Hachette. 2003.

FRICKER, J. *Le guide du bien maigrir.* Odile Jacob, 1993.

MONTIGNAC, M. *Savoir gérer son alimentation ou comment maigrir en faisant des repas d'affaires.* Artulen, 1989.

NOEL, A. *Les sauces diététiques.* Ed Saep, 1990.

RICHE, D. *L'alimentation du sportif en 80 questions.* Vigot, 2002.

SHELTON, H., J. WILLARD, J. OSWALD. *The Original Natural Hygiene Weight Loss Diet Book.* 1968.

SHELTON, H. *Les combinaisons alimentaires et votre santé.* Le courrier du livre, 1968.

SMOLLER and COLL. *Popular and very low calories in the treatment of obesity.* Aspen Publications, 1988.

STORA, J.-B. *Quand le corps prend la relève.* Odile Jacob, 2000.

VALERIE, ANNE. *Le grand livre de la cuisine légère à la maison.* Succès du livre, 1986.

WAYSFELD, B. *Le poids et le moi.* Armand Colin, 2003.

WEIGHT WATCHERS. *Le nouveau livre gourmand.* Belfond, 1993.

ZERMATI, J.-P. *La fin des régimes.* Hachette, 1998.

Articles:

ALBERT, K.G.M.M., F.A. GRIES. *Management of non-insulin dependant diabetes mellitus in Europe: a consensus view.* Diabetic Med, 1988; 5: 275-81.

AMATRUDA and COLL. *Vigorous supplementation of a hypocaloric diet prevents cardiac arrythmias and mineral depletion.* Am J Med, 74 : 1016, 1983.

APFELBAUM, M., and COLL. *Low and very low calorie diets.* Am J Clin Nutr., (suppl.) 45: 1126, 1987.

APFELBAUM, M., J. BOSTARRON, D. LACATIS. *Effects of calorie restriction and excessive caloric intake on energy expenditure.* Am J Clin Nutr., 24: 1405-1409,1971.

BALKAU, B., M.A. CHARLES and the European Group for the Study of Insulin Resistance (EGIR). *Frequency of the WHO metabolic syndrome in European cohorts, and an alternative definition of an insulin resistance syndrome.* Diabetes Metab., 2002 28: 364-76.

BLACKBURN, G.L., P.G. LIDNER. *Multidisciplinary approach to obesity utilizing fasting by protein-sparing therapy.* Obesity Bariatric Med., Vol. 5 No. 6, 1976: 198-216.

BLACKBURN, PALGI and COLL. *Multidisciplinary treatment of obesity with a protein-sparing modified fast.* Am J Public Health, 75: 1190-1985.

CONSEIL SUPERIEUR DU DIABETE. *Diabète sucré : prise en charge, traitement et recherche en Europe.* La Déclaration de St-Vincent et son Programme. (Adaptation française par le Conseil Supérieur du Diabète). Diabète Metab., 1992, 18 : 329-77.

JENKINS, D.J.A. *Dietary carbohydrates and their glycemic responses.* Jama 21: 2829-2831, 1984.

MC CARTH, M.F. *A paradox resolved: the postprandial model of insulin resistance explains why gynoid adiposity appears to be protective.* Med. Hypotheses 2003; 61 (12): 173-6.

RAISON, J. *Le syndrome métabolique, une définition pas si vague.* Nutritions et facteurs de risque, nov. 2003, n° 1, 22-24.

TCHERNOF, A., E.T. POEHLMAN, J.P. DESPRES. *Body fat distribution, the menopause transition and hormone replacement therapy.* Diabetes Metab. 2000; 26: 12-20.

VAGUE, P. *Aspects cliniques et thérapeutiques : reconnaître et traiter le syndrome polymétabolique.* Nutritions et facteurs de risque, nov. 2003, n° 1, 25-29.

VERMEULEN, A. *Effects of a short-term (4 weeks) protein-sparing modified fast on plasma lipids and lipoproteins in obese women.* Metabolism. Jul. 1996, 45 (7): 908-14.

VINDREAU, C., D. GINESTAT. *Boulimie sucrée, boulimie salée, profils émotionnels et statut pondéral.* L'Encéphale, 1989, n° 15, 233-38.